Cardiac Ultrasound

Leonard M Shapiro
BSc, MD, FRCP, FACC
Consultant Cardiologist
Papworth and Addenbrookes Hospital
Cambridge

Antoinette Kenny
MD, MRCPI, MRCP(UK)
Consultant Cardiologist
Freeman Hospital
Newcastle upon Tyne

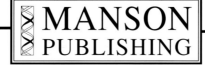

MANSON
PUBLISHING

Copyright © 1998 Manson Publishing Ltd
ISBN 1–874545–08–1

A CIP catalogue record for this book is available from the British Library.

For full details of all Manson Publishing Ltd titles please write to
Manson Publishing Ltd, 73 Corringham Road, London NW11 7DL, UK.

Design and layout: The Little Round Consultancy
Text editing: William Down
Project Management: John Ormiston
Colour reproduction: Tenon & Polert Colour Scanning Ltd., HK
Printed by: Dah Hua Printing Press Co. Ltd, Hong Kong

CONTENTS

FOREWORD

The quality of ultrasound imaging, both for tissue structure and in Doppler methods, has evolved rapidly. To help interpret the images and patient findings, simple, short, and efficient ways to review and compare these with illustrative examples and tables of diagnostic criteria and observations are needed. The most useful presentation is a resource book that is easy to use and of high quality. However, many of the textbooks in echocardiography, definitive and detailed as they are, have so expanded to cover the variety of technologies used and the detailed interplay of methods and observations that they are no longer particularly helpful as quick references.

The present work, *Cardiac Ultrasound*, by Drs Shapiro and Kenny from Cambridge, UK, and Newcastle, UK, respectively, is a pictorial reference that draws upon the authors' experience to provide useful tips, hallmark observations, and pitfalls in clinical echocardiography. It includes transthoracic and transesophageal findings as necessary, depending on which of the two methods is usually used for definitive diagnosis. Helpful diagrams accompany the didactic echocardiograms and are, as the authors hope and have expressed in the Preface, useful not only for physicians and those in cardiology training but also for technicians who study and perform echocardiography.

An atlas of two-dimensional anatomy of the heart that a colleague and I prepared in 1980–1981 was in great demand at that time and, although it is now technologically obsolete, the drawings are still used by many. I believe that to have a high quality, up-to-date graphic reference for state-of-the-art echocardiography is helpful to many physicians involved in the field and I commend the authors on their efforts, as I commend their efforts to you the reader.

David J. Sahn, MD
Director, The Clinical Care Center for Congenital
Heart Disease
Professor of Pediatrics, Diagnostic Radiology, and
Obstetrics & Gynecology
Oregon Health Sciences University
Portland, Oregon
USA

PREFACE

The development of ultrasound imaging of the heart has had a dramatic impact in clinical cardiology. Its ability to provide immediate, non-invasive diagnostic information has obviated the need for invasive studies in many patients and, as a portable and relatively inexpensive technique, it competes favorably with more expensive imaging modalities. The technology has advanced considerably from the earliest stages of M-mode recordings, the progress being one of gradual evolution with occasional great advances. Even in those early days the application of ultrasound to patients with valvular and myocardial disease was obvious, but with the parallel advances in computer technology a diverse array of diagnostic ultrasound techniques have become available.

The sonographer's diagnostic armamentarium now includes techniques of transesophageal, intravascular and stress echocardiography. Transesophageal echocardiography, in particular, has had a unique impact as it enables imaging of cardiac structures not readily accessible from the transthoracic approach, while it overcomes the problem of poor acoustic windows. There are many developments in ultrasound waiting in the wings, which may lead to future improvements in imaging and data interpretation.

Both the authors have much experience in echocardiography, LMS being the founder president of the British Society of Echocardiography. Both are Directors of Echocardiographic Services at their respective Regional Cardiothoracic centers, which provide state-of-the-art cardiac ultrasound services, including training of medical and technical staff in these techniques. This book is based on the authors own practical experience and is aimed at physicians, physicians-in-training and technical staff involved in the management of patients who have cardiac disease.

In addition to being a pictorial reference for all those involved in performing cardiac ultrasound, this book also draws on the teaching expertise of the authors to provide the reader with useful tips for the improvement of technical skills, to highlight pitfalls in interpretation for the unwary and to emphasize the interpretation of imaging data within clinical context. All varieties of ultrasound imaging in use in a modern echocardiographic laboratory are described, including multiplane transesophageal echocardiography, stress echocardiography and intraoperative and intravascular imaging.

Although further technical developments are anticipated, these will require a basic understanding and practical competence in the range of facilities already available. We feel that now is an ideal time to consolidate present knowledge so as to appreciate fully advances that may be ahead. We therefore believe that the timing of publication of this book is appropriate for all those involved in echocardiographic practice.

Leonard M. Shapiro

Antoinette Kenny

Acknowledgments

We are indebted to the many friends and colleagues who have contributed to this text. We particularly thank our technicians without whose skilled help little would have been achieved.

Addenbrookes Hospital: Helen Murfet.
Freeman Hospital: Joanne Forster, Barry Cumberledge, Christine Cummins, Julie Schuster.
Papworth Hospital: Christopher Wisbey, Anita Gebbels, Dinah Shore.

Abbreviations

A arch	Aortic arch	LVPW	Left ventricular posterior wall
AO	Aorta	MPA	Main pulmonary artery
AoV	Aortic valve	MRI	Magnetic resonance imaging
ASV	Aortic stroke volume	MV	Mitral valve
AVS	Anterior ventricular septum	PA	Pulmonary artery
CT	Computed tomography	PISA	Proximal isovelocity surface area
DAO	Descending aorta	PSV	Pulmonary stoke volume
IAS	Intra-atrial septum	RA	Right atrium
IVC	Inferior vena cava	RPA	Right pulmonary artery
IVS	Interventricular septum	RV	Right ventricle
IVUS	Intravascular ultrasound	RVOT	Right ventricle outflow tract
LA	Left atrium	SEP	Systolic ejection period
LAA	Left atrial appendage	SVC	Superior vena cava
LPA	Left pulmonary artery	TEE	Transesophageal echocardiography
LV	Left ventricle	TV	Tricuspid valve
LVH	Left ventricular hypertrophy	VSD	Ventricular septal defect
LVOT	Left ventricular outflow tract	VTI	Velocity time integral

BASIC PHYSICS

Sound travels in waves. Frequency, the number of waves per unit time, is measured in Hertz (Hz) with 1 Hz representing 1 cycle per second. The wavelength is inversely proportional to the frequency. Ultrasound is high frequency sound waves above the range that is detected by the human ear. Frequencies of 1.5–7.5 MHz are used in echocardiography and the wavelength at 1.5 MHz is approximately 1.0 mm. The speed of sound in soft tissues such as the heart is 1540 m/s. There is a trade-off between transducer frequency and penetration; higher frequency sound waves give better resolution, but have poor penetration. In adult echocardiography, therefore, a lower frequency transducer is used, which allows imaging of deep structures; higher frequency transducers are used more for pediatric imaging.

When ultrasound travels through tissue, a certain proportion is reflected back to the transducer at interfaces between tissues of different acoustic impedance such as the interface between blood and heart valves or myocardial tissue. Ultrasound is generated by the piezoelectric effect. An electrical charge is applied across a piezoelectric crystal. This causes deformation of the crystal, which oscillates at a predetermined frequency which is dependent on its thickness. To image the heart through the relatively small acoustic windows, a transducer which creates a fan of ultrasound and sector-shaped image is employed. The ultrasound fan typically contains 120 scan lines, each of which is produced by sending a pulse down that line; the reflected echos from that line are then collected. The same transducer is used both to transmit and to receive the ultrasound.

A mechanical or electronic method may be used to steer ultrasound pulses down the individual scan lines. Mechanical transducers employ either rotating or oscillatory systems. Electronic beam steering is achieved using phased array technology. The crystal element of the transducer is divided into 64 or 128 individual elements, each with its own electronic connection. Each element is fired and the individual wavefronts merge to form a compound wave. Steering direction is determined by the sequence in which elements are fired. Phased array technology is more reliable than mechanical as the beam is steered without using moving parts; it also allows superior beam focusing. A disadvantage of phased array transducers is the near field artifact caused by 'side lobes' which are off-axis ultrasound beams formed by interaction between individual elements. Annular array transducers combine features of both mechanical and phased array technology. The beam is steered mechanically but individual elements are fired in sequence as in phased array transducers which allows narrow beam formation and improved resolution.

Principles of Doppler

Doppler echocardiography is based on the Doppler effect, first described by the Austrian physicist Johann Doppler in 1842. The principle describes the change in frequency in sound waves caused by the motion of the source or the observer. In cross-sectional echocardiography, we are interested in sound waves reflected from boundaries of solid structures such as the walls of cavities, the valves, and pericardium. In Doppler echocardiography, the interest is in sound reflected back from red blood cells. The frequency of sound reflected back from red blood cells is compared to that of emitted sound. The difference in frequency between emitted and returning ultrasound is the 'Doppler shift'. If the reflected sound has a higher frequency than the emitted sound, the Doppler shift is positive and this signifies flow towards the transducer. If the reflected sound is lower in frequency, it is termed a negative Doppler shift, and represents flow away from the transducer. The Doppler equation relates the Doppler shift to the velocity of red blood cell flow:

$$\Delta f = \frac{2fv \cos \theta}{c}$$

Δf = Doppler shift
f = frequency of transmitted sound
v = velocity of red blood cells
θ = angle between blood flow and direction of ultrasound beam
c = velocity of sound

The direction of ultrasound must therefore be parallel to the direction of blood flow for measurement of absolute blood velocity. Lesser degrees of alignment will result in underestimation of velocity.

Spectral Doppler display uses variations in gray scale to indicate different intensities in returned

Doppler signals according to the number of red blood cells travelling at each velocity. Flow towards the transducer is, by convention, displayed above a horizontal axis and flow away from the transducer is shown below the line. There are three modes of Doppler currently in use: pulsed Doppler, continuous-wave Doppler, and color-flow mapping.

In pulsed Doppler the transducer alternates between emitting and receiving pulses of ultrasound. Blood flow at a specific area of the heart can be examined by placing a sample volume at that site. The transducer emits a pulse and then waits for the returning signals from that site before transmitting the next pulse. The equipment is calibrated to analyze ultrasound returning only from that area of interest. The maximum velocity that can be detected by pulsed Doppler is limited, as velocities are sampled by pulses rather than continuously. The Nyquist limit is a term which defines the maximum velocity that can be measured. Measurement of frequency shift and hence velocities requires a pulse repetition rate of at least twice the Doppler frequency shift of the sampled area. If the Nyquist limit is exceeded, then the phenomenon of aliasing occurs. The sampling rate is too low to detect the high velocity, which is cut off and displayed in the opposite direction on the spectral display. Aliasing may occur to an extent where high velocities are wrapped around the display several times. The Nyquist limit is dependent on the pulse repetition frequency (higher when the sample volume is nearer the transducer and the distance for ultrasound to travel is less) and the frequency of the transducer. Aliasing will occur at higher velocities for lower frequency transducers.

In continuous-wave Doppler the transducer has two elements, one continuously emitting ultrasound and the other continuously detecting the reflected sound waves. The pulse repetition frequency, therefore, is infinite and there is no limit on the velocity which can be measured. However, as velocities are measured along the whole length of the beam there is no spatial resolution.

Pulsed and continuous-wave Doppler are complementary techniques. Pulsed Doppler allows high spatial resolution, but cannot measure high velocities. It is better for discriminating between laminar and turbulent flow as the spectral trace is narrow, whereas with continuous-wave Doppler velocities are measured along the length of the beam and there is spectral broadening. Continuous-wave Doppler can measure high velocities, but there is no spatial resolution. In normal hearts most blood flow velocities are <1.5 m/s and can be measured by pulsed Doppler. In disease states velocities are often high and continuous-wave Doppler techniques are necessary.

Color flow mapping may be superimposed on cross-sectional or M-mode images. It is a pulsed Doppler technique where blood velocity and direction data are sampled down a number of scan lines The various velocities are color-coded and displayed by velocity and direction in relation to the transducer. Normal flow towards the transducer is depicted as dull shades of red, with normal flow away from the transducer in blue. As it is a pulsed Doppler technique it has the same limitation in terms of inability to measure high velocities as pulsed Doppler. When aliasing occurs the colors become brighter and a mosaic appearance occurs.

2 THE NORMAL HEART

Standard Transthoracic Imaging Planes

Although there is an infinite number of possible imaging planes The American Society of Echocardiography has defined a series of standardized imaging views. These standard imaging planes are designated on the basis of:
- Transducer location.
- Spatial orientation of the imaging plane.
- Structures recorded.

They employ parasternal, apical, subcostal and suprasternal windows. In **1** the transducer positions employed in echocardiography are illustrated diagrammatically.

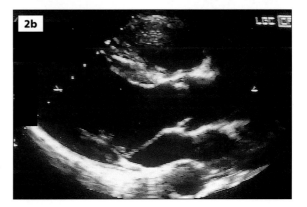

Parasternal long-axis images with corresponding line drawings

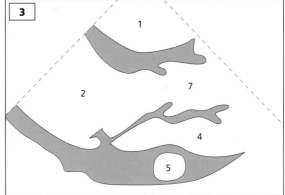

The parasternal long axis view of the left heart is obtained by placing the transducer on the left sternal edge, choosing an intercostal space that will align the interventricular septum perpendicular to the transducer. This plane transects the heart from the aortic root through both leaflets of the mitral valve and the body of the left ventricle. This plane is ideally suited to evaluate the anterior right ventricular free wall and right ventricular cavity, the aortic root, aortic valve, left atrium, mitral valve, and body of the left ventricle, but not the apex. The function of the anterobasal portion of the interventricular

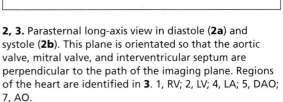

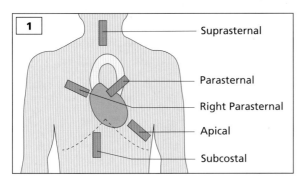

1. Transducer positions to obtain parasternal, apical, subcostal, and suprasternal echo images.

2, 3. Parasternal long-axis view in diastole (**2a**) and systole (**2b**). This plane is orientated so that the aortic valve, mitral valve, and interventricular septum are perpendicular to the path of the imaging plane. Regions of the heart are identified in **3**. 1, RV; 2, LV; 4, LA; 5, DAO; 7, AO.

septum and posterior wall may be observed. This view is unsuitable for quantitative Doppler examination of mitral valve flow and left ventricular outflow as the Doppler beam is perpendicular to the direction of flow. Mitral and aortic regurgitation however may be detected, as the regurgitant jets may be eccentric.

Parasternal long axis views of the right ventricular inflow and outflow tracts are obtained as described in **4** and **5**.

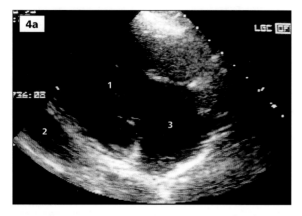

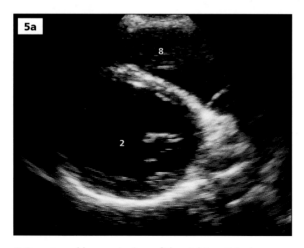

4. Parasternal long-axis view of the right ventricular inflow tract. This is obtained by angling medially and inferiorly from the parasternal long axis view. This view is particularly useful for evaluating tricuspid valve structure and function (**4b**). 1, RV; 2, LV; 3, RA.

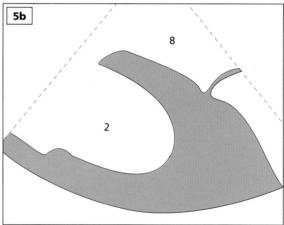

5. Parasternal long-axis view of the right ventricular outflow tract. Lateral and superior angulation of the transducer from the parasternal long-axis view will produce an image of the long axis of the right ventricular outflow tract, pulmonary valve and main pulmonary artery. Regions of the heart are identified in **5b**. 2, LV; 8, RVOT.

Parasternal short-axis images with corresponding line drawings

Parasternal short-axis views are orientated at a 90° angle to the long-axis plane by clockwise rotation of the transducer. There are three standard short-axis views, which are obtained at the levels of the aortic valve, the mitral valve and the papillary muscles.

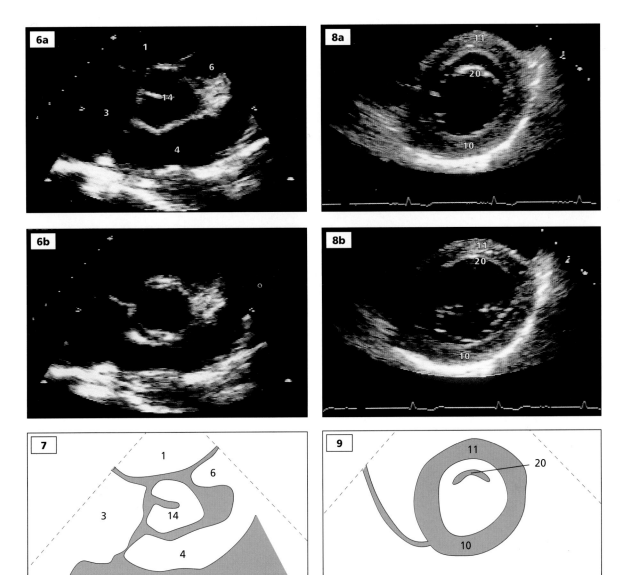

6, 7. Parasternal short-axis view of the aortic valve; diastole (**6a**) showing the right coronary and non-coronary commissure and systole (**6b**) with the aortic valve open. This imaging plane is best for assessment of aortic valve leaflets; sinuses of Valsalva; examination of the left atrium; and the interatrial septum. It is also the primary view for assessing the relative positions of the great vessels. The tricuspid and pulmonary valves may be well-visualized and their function assessed. The architecture of the heart is illustrated in **7**. 1, RV; 3, RA; 4, LA; 6, PA; 14, AoV.

8, 9. Parasternal short-axis view of the mitral valve. This is ideal for directly planimetering the mitral valve orifice in mitral stenosis. As the left ventricular cavity and walls are well seen and this view is equivalent to the M-mode position, it is useful for measuring left ventricular cavity and wall thickness. In diastole (**8a**) the mitral valve is seen open and in (**8b**) parts of the closed mitral valve are seen. Fragments of the tricuspid valve may be seen. The architecture of the heart is illustrated in **9**. 10, LVPW; 11, IVS; 20, MV.

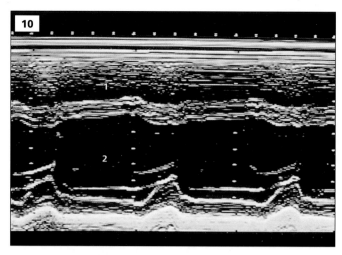

10. An M-mode echocardiogram taken through the upper left ventricle. The M-mode recording is a graph of echos down a single scan line against time. All M-mode recordings are made from the parasternal window. The M-mode beam must cross cardiac structures perpendicularly, and the left ventricular recording is achieved by placing the beam just below the tips of the mitral valve leaflets. Recordings at this level are used for measuring left ventricular internal dimensions and myocardial wall thickness. Parameters of left ventricular function and mass such as ejection fraction, fractional shortening, and left ventricular mass may be derived from this recording. The posterior wall is seen anterior to the fibrous (dense) pericardium. 1, RV; 2, LV.

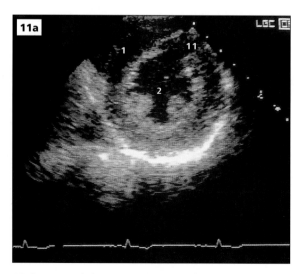

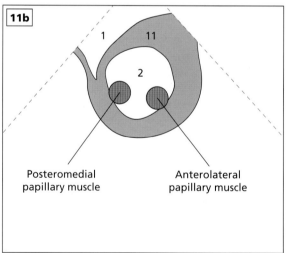

Posteromedial papillary muscle

Anterolateral papillary muscle

11. Parasternal short-axis view at papillary muscle level (systolic frame). The circular left ventricle is recorded in the center of the sector and a small portion of the right ventricle is displayed anteriorly and to the left. The posteromedial papillary muscle is displayed to the left and the anterolateral papillary muscle to the right. Ventricular septal defects may be identified from this plane. This view displays territories supplied by all three main epicardial coronary arteries. **11b** illustrates the heart structures.) 1, RV; 2, LV; 11, IVS.

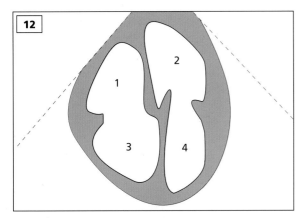

Apical views with corresponding line drawings

These views are recorded with the transducer located over the cardiac apex with the imaging plane directed toward the base of the heart.

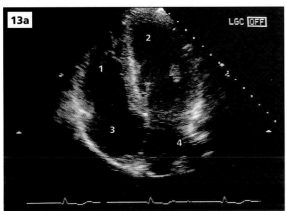

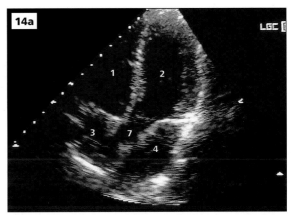

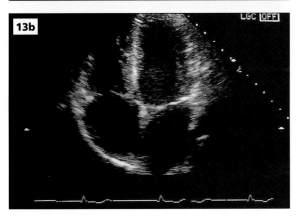

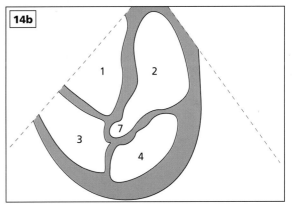

12, 13. Apical four-chamber view. The left ventricular apex is well visualized. This orientation permits optimal visualization of mitral and tricuspid valve leaflets. The tricuspid valve is inserted into the ventricular septum nearer the apex than the mitral valve. In this view the Doppler beam is aligned with flow through the valves and it is the plane best suited for assessment of stenosis and regurgitation of the mitral and tricuspid valves. The atria are well-visualized and the pulmonary veins may be seen entering the left atrium. The imaging beam is parallel to the atrial and ventricular septae, making this view less ideal for detecting septal defects. The septal and lateral left ventricular walls and the right ventricular free wall are imaged. 1, RV; 2, LV; 3, RA; 4, LA.

14. Apical five-chamber view. Anterior angulation of the transducer from the apical four-chamber plane is used to visualize the aortic valve and root (fifth chamber) in addition to the other four chambers. This allows assessment of left ventricular outflow and aortic regurgitation (right anterior oblique equivalent). 1, RV; 2, LV; 3, RA; 4, LA; 7, AO.

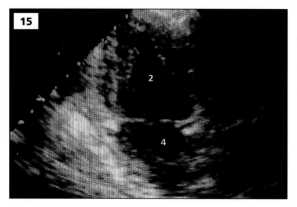

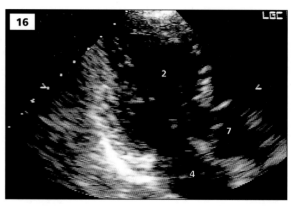

15. Rotation of the transducer 90° anticlockwise from the four-chamber position produces the apical two-chamber view which is used for assessment of systolic function. This view images the inferior and anterior left ventricular walls. 2, LV; 4, LA.

16. Apical long-axis view. This is similar in orientation to the parasternal long-axis view of the left ventricle, but is recorded from the cardiac apex. It is useful for recording aortic flow. 2, LV; 4, LA; 7, AO.

Subcostal views with corresponding line drawings

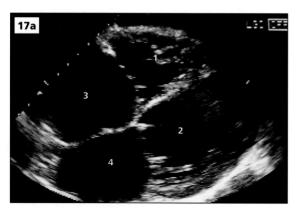

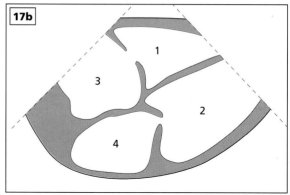

17. Subcostal long-axis view. This is useful for examining the right side of the heart, and in particular the interatrial and interventricular septae. The septae are oriented perpendicular to the scan plane in this view and therefore echo dropout does not occur. It may also be the best view for imaging free right ventricular wall and free lateral left ventricular wall motion. The architecture of the heart is also shown in **17b**. 1, RV; 2, LV; 3, RA; 4, LA.

It is essential to learn the standard imaging planes, but to obtain the maximum information from the study experienced sonographers use off-axis views in addition to the standard ones.

Suprasternal views with corresponding line drawings

These views are particularly useful for examining the aortic arch.

> The recognition of a normal echocardiogram requires practice and experience. It is often more apparent to the operator that the scan is normal than to those reporting at a later date.

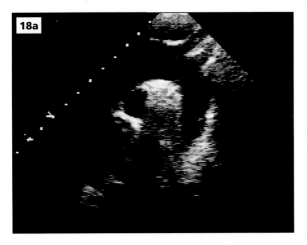

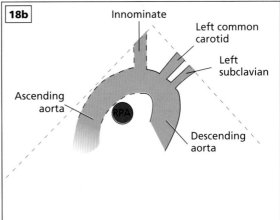

18. This long-axis view illustrates the ascending portion of the aorta, the arch and the descending aorta. The left carotid and left subclavian branches of the aortic arch are also visible. The left atrium is behind the right pulmonary artery (RPA).

Normal Doppler echocardiography

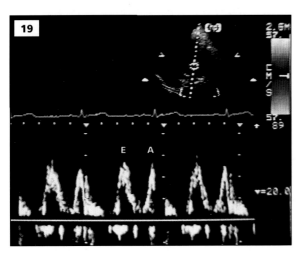

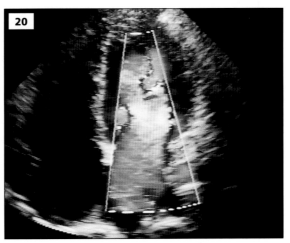

19. Normal mitral flow assessed by pulsed Doppler from the apex. Flow through the mitral valve in diastole is towards the transducer, and therefore displayed above the line. The velocity spectrum is M-shaped. The initial peak (E) represents passive flow in early diastole from left atrium to left ventricle. The second, smaller peak represents increased flow in late diastole from atrial contraction (A). The peak velocity is <1 m/s in normal mitral valves and the clean spectral envelope indicates that flow is laminar.

20. Color flow map from the apex depicting flow in diastole through a normal mitral valve. As flow is towards the transducer and laminar it is displayed in dull shades of red.

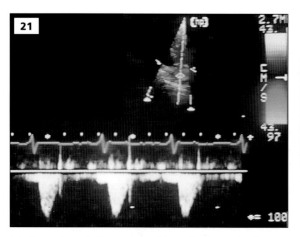

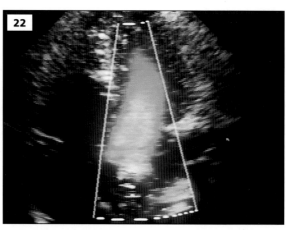

21. Normal aortic flow assessed by pulsed Doppler from the apex. Flow through the aortic valve is away from the transducer and displayed below the line. Flow is laminar and in this example is just >1 m/s.

22. Color-flow map from the apex with systolic flow passing from the left ventricle through a normal aortic valve and away from the transducer displayed in dull shades of blue.

Transesophageal Echocardiography

Transesophageal echocardiography is the study of the heart from the esophagus and is achieved by mounting a small transducer on the tip of a flexible endoscope. The close apposition of the esophagus to the posterior surface of the heart overcomes access problems associated with transthoracic imaging and allows the use of higher-frequency transducers, thereby improving image quality. Transesophageal probe technology has progressed from monoplane and biplane imaging to multiplane transducers. Monoplane imaging utilizes a single transducer to obtain transverse cuts of the heart. Biplane imaging has a second transducer mounted at a 90° angle to the horizontal plane for longitudinal imaging. The multiplane probe provides up to 360° window by electronically rotating the transducer. Transesophageal echocardiography is the imaging procedure of choice for investigation of infective endocarditis, prosthetic valve function, cardiac masses, selected native valve disease, diseases of the thoracic aorta, and detection of cardiac sources of emboli.

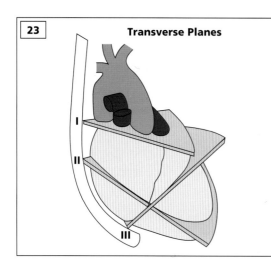

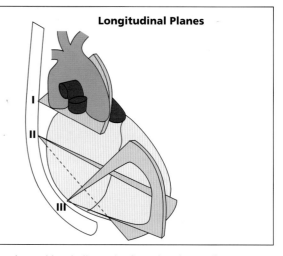

23. This illustrates diagrammatically the three basic transverse and longitudinal scanning planes for complete examination of the heart. Position I obtains images of the basal cardiovascular structures, position II at the mid-esophageal level allows the four-chamber and two-chamber views, and position III provides transgastric views.

Standard imaging planes
Esophageal views
Basal views

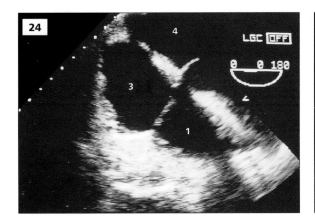

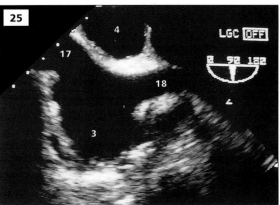

24, 25. The atrial septum is shown imaged in transverse (**24**) and longitudinal (**25**) planes. The longitudinal plane at this level images the inferior and superior vena cavae entering the right atrium. It is particularly useful for detecting a sinus venosus atrial septal defect. I, RV; 3, RA; 4, LA; 17, IVC; 18, SVC.

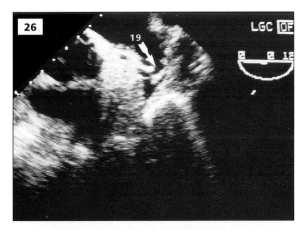

26. In the transverse plane, and by raising the transducer higher in the esophagus, rotation to the left of the patient and anteflexion will image the left atrial appendage. The proximal coronary arteries may also be imaged at this level. The left atrial appendage may be multilobar and should be examined in more than one plane. 19, LAA.

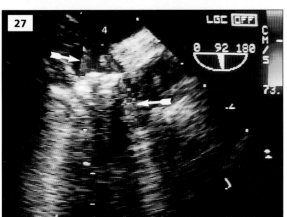

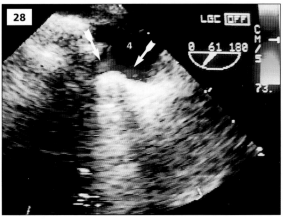

27, 28. The normal upper and lower left (**27**) and right (**28**) pulmonary veins are imaged by color-flow mapping just above the level of the atrial appendage. The pulmonary veins are often best seen in the longitudinal plane (arrows). 4, LA.

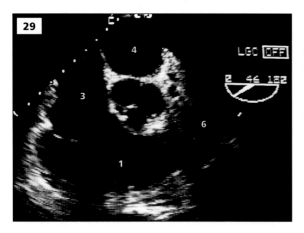

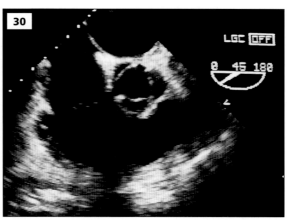

29, 30 Advancing further into the esophagus, a multiplane probe imaging at approximately 45° produces a true short axis of the aortic valve in diastole (**29**) and systole (**30**) with clear imaging of each cusp. This is superior to the standard transverse plane for the assessment of the aortic valve. 1, RV; 3, RA; 4, LA; 6, PA.

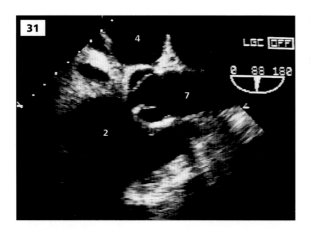

31. Rotation to the longitudinal plane at this level will image the ascending aorta. This longitudinal view is particularly useful when examining for vegetations, and the ascending aorta for dissection. 2, LV; 4, LA; 7, AO.

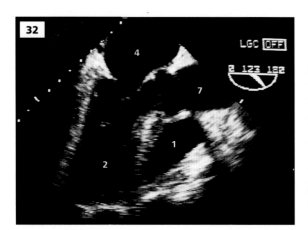

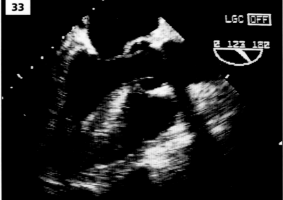

32 (diastole) and **33** (systole). The 120° image at this level facilitates detection of aortic regurgitation and allows examination of the subaortic area for obstruction in hypertrophic cardiomyopathy and subvalvular aortic stenosis. 1, RV; 2, LV; 4, LA; 7, AO.

Lower esophageal views

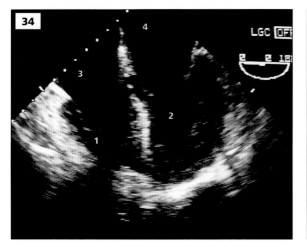

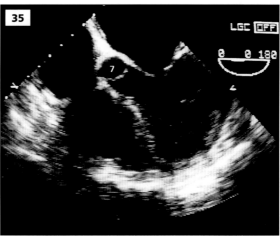

34. Four-chamber view transverse plane. The anterior and posterior leaflets of the mitral valve are readily seen in this diastolic frame. This view allows assessment of mitral and tricuspid regurgitation and Doppler assessment of transmitral flow. 1, RV; 2, LV; 3, RA; 4, LA.

35. Slight anteflexion of the probe from the four-chamber transverse plane produces the five-chamber view, which is useful for detecting aortic regurgitation. 7, AO.

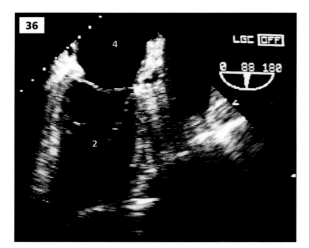

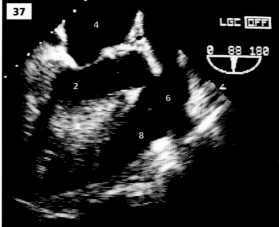

36. Rotation at this level to approximately 90° produces the two-chamber longitudinal view of the left atrium, left ventricle, and mitral valve. This view images the anterior and inferior left ventricular walls, whereas the transverse plane four-chamber view images the septal and lateral walls. It is often superior for detecting mitral regurgitation, particularly in mitral prostheses. Slight angulation of the probe will produce good views of the left atrial appendage. 2, LV; 4, LA.

37. Rotating the probe to the patient's right will give a long axis view of the right ventricular outflow tract with aortic and pulmonary valves. Slight withdrawal of the probe images the main pulmonary artery to the level of bifurcation. 2, LV; 4, LA; 6, PA; 8, RVOT.

Gastric views

Transgastric views are obtained by passing the probe into the fundus of the stomach and employing anteflexion to maintain contact.

The degree of probe advancement and anteflexion determines the structures imaged. Greater anteflexion gives images toward the base of the heart, with views of the mitral and tricuspid valves; lesser anteflexion displays the mid and apical regions of the ventricles. The imaging plane is then steered from transverse to longitudinal views.

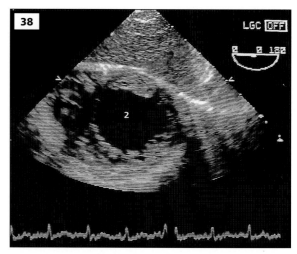

38. Transgastric transverse plane at mid-papillary level, diastolic frame. This view facilitates cross-sectional evaluation of left ventricular function. 2, LV.

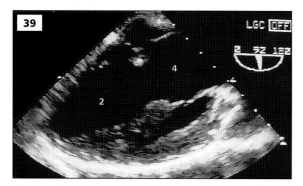

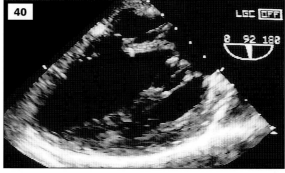

39, 40. The transgastric longitudinal imaging plane displays the left ventricle and left atrium in a foreshortened apical view. Both leaflets of the mitral valve, the papillary muscles and chordae are seen.

Diastolic (**39**) and systolic (**40**) frames demonstrate left ventricular contraction from base to apex. This view is particularly useful for the assessment of the subvalvular structures. 2, LV; 4, LA.

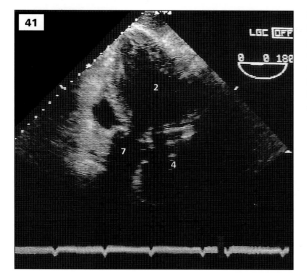

41. Lowering the probe further into the stomach and maintaining considerable anteflexion produces a four- and five-chamber view in the transverse plane. This distal view is particularly useful for Doppler interrogation of the aortic and pulmonary valves as it allows correct alignment of the Doppler beam with both left and right ventricular outflow. It also allows assessment of the ventricular side of mitral prostheses. 2, LV; 4, LA; 7, AO.

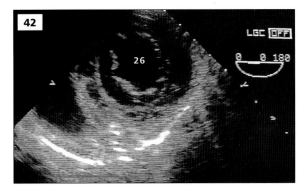

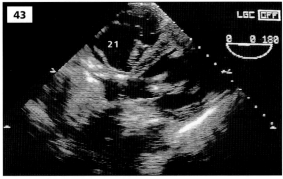

42. As the probe is raised to the level of the diaphragm a short-axis view of the mitral valve in the transverse plane is obtained, and direct planimetry of the mitral orifice (26) can be performed.

43. Slight rotation to the patient's right will demonstrate a short-axis view of the tricuspid valve. 21, TV.

Thoracic aorta

In the lower esophagus the probe is rotated 180° to image the descending thoracic aorta. The transverse plane yields cross-sectional round slices of the aorta (**44**), whereas the longitudinal plane provides long axis images of the tube (**45**). As the probe is raised to approximately 25 cm from the mouth, the aortic arch appears in view (**46**). Rotation of the probe to the right will image the transverse and ascending aorta. There is a small blind spot in the ascending aorta where the trachea is interposed between the esophagus and ascending aorta. The longitudinal plane will minimize this ultrasonic blind spot.

> *Transesophageal echocardiography has revolutionized echocardiography, as not only can structures unobtainable by transthoracic echocardiography be imaged, but transesophageal echocardiography should be used when images are suboptimal.*

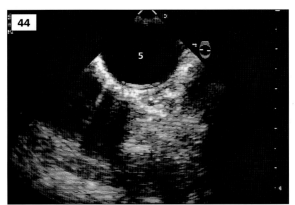

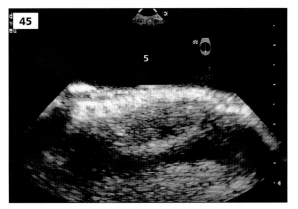

44–46. Imaging the descending thoracic aorta and arch (see text for description). 5, DAO; 22, A arch.

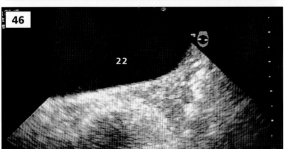

Normal Variants

An inadequate echocardiographic window or off-axis imaging may produce alterations in the appearance of normal cardiac structures. This situation is usually readily recognized.

Normal variants and congenital structures may simulate pathologic intracardiac masses. The atria and interatrial septum contain many such structures which may pose diagnostic problems and are better visualized by transesophageal echocardiography.

Right atrium

The eustachian valve is a vestigial structure which in fetal life directs blood flow from the inferior vena cava across the fossa ovalis. A persistent eustachian valve is seen by transesophageal echocardiography in up to 25% of adults.

The Chiari network is a remnant of the embryonic sinus venosus and is found in 2–3% of normal hearts at autopsy. This normal variant is seldom of clinical importance and echocardiographically appears as a filamentous membranous network in the right atrium with characteristic chaotic mobility.

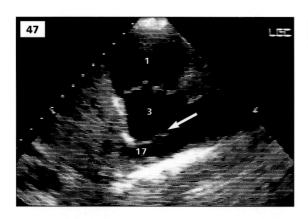

47. A prominent eustachian valve is seen (arrow) as a horizontal linear echo arising from the anterior margin of the orifice of the inferior vena cava in this parasternal long-axis right ventricular inflow view. 1, RV; 3, RA; 17, IVC.

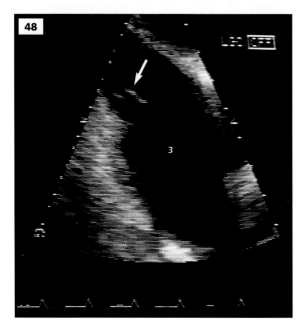

48. In this transesophageal right ventricular inflow view (longitudinal plane) the eustachian valve (arrow) can be clearly seen as a thin filamentous structure at the junction of the inferior vena cava with the right atrium. The mobility of this flap may be appreciated by serial frames. Color flow Doppler will demonstrate that there is no obstruction from this structure. 3, RA.

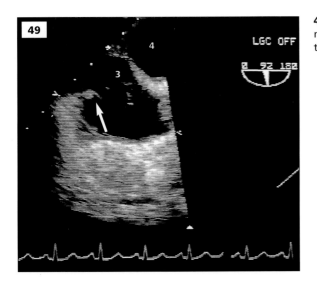

49. A large and mobile eustachian valve (arrow) may be mistaken for a Chiari network, vegetation, thrombus or tumor. 3, RA; 4, LA.

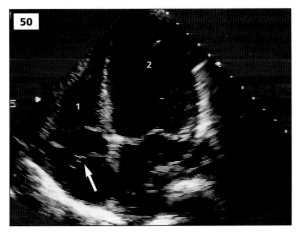

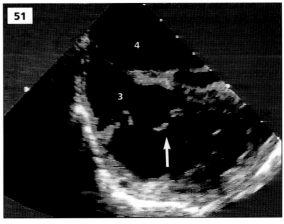

50, 51. Apical four-chamber view illustrating a mass of echos behind the tricuspid valve consistent with the complex appearance of the Chiari network (arrow). The mobility and undulation of the network with blood flow can be seen in this transesophageal transverse view. 1, RV; 2, LV; 3, RA; 4, LA.

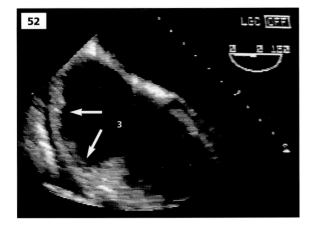

52. At transesophageal echocardiography the normal right atrial wall demonstrates small ridges and elevations consistent with pectinate muscles (arrows). These are multiple, have the same density as the underlying tissue, and may thicken during atrial contraction – all of which help to distinguish them from thrombi. 3, RA.

Left atrium

The left atrial appendage is rarely seen adequately by transthoracic echocardiography, but is visualized well by transesophageal imaging, which is therefore used to interrogate the appendage for thrombus (see 334, 335).

The normal left atrial appendage is lined by small pectinate muscle ridges that must be distinguished from small thrombi. Left atrial appendage pectinate muscles are usually multiple and have the same density as underlying tissue. The septum between the left atrial appendage and upper left pulmonary vein may have a bulbous dense tip which should not be mistaken for a thrombus or other mass.

Interatrial septum

An interatrial septal aneurysm is a congenital aneurysmal formation of the atrial septum, typically involving the region of the fossa ovalis. Echocardiographically it appears as a prominent linear bulge arising from the interatrial septum which, by definition, should involve at least a 1.5 cm length of the septum and swing at least 1.1 cm into either atrium, or have a total excursion of 1.1 cm. In general, the interatrial septal aneurysm demonstrates phasic motion with respiration and swings into the right atrium with a Valsalva maneuver. Recently, interest in such aneurysms has increased as they have been implicated as a potential cardiac source of emboli. This may be related to the formation of thrombus within the aneurysm, or the frequent association of an interatrial septal aneurysm with a patent foramen ovale.

Contrast injections are more sensitive than color-flow Doppler alone in detecting a patent foramen ovale. Agitated saline is injected into a peripheral vein, forming microbubbles which opacify the right atrium. A Valsalva maneuver may accentuate the flow.

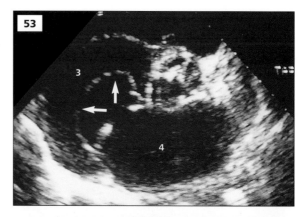

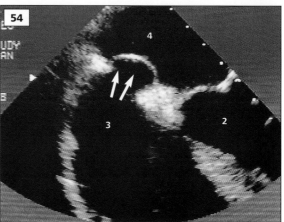

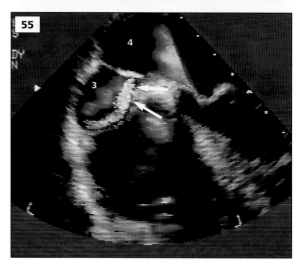

53–55. Parasternal short-axis views at the level of the aortic valve, illustrating a large atrial septal aneurysm bulging into the right atrium (arrows). In this example there is a residual atrial septal defect (**53**). In this transverse plane transesophageal image an atrial septal aneurysm (arrows) is seen to bulge into the left atrium (**54**). Color-flow Doppler shows a jet of turbulent flow (arrows) from left to right atrium through an associated patent foramen ovale (**55**). 2, LV; 3, RA; 4, LA.

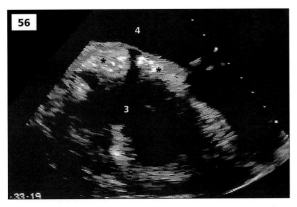

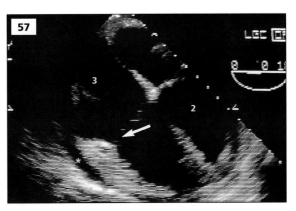

56. Lipomatous hypertrophy of the interatrial septum is characterized by the accumulation of excessive adipose tissue in the interatrial septum. This produces a characteristic thickening of the interatrial septum (*) which spares the fossa ovalis, giving a bi-lobed or dumb-bell shape as seen in this four-chamber transverse plane transesophageal view. 3, RA; 4, LA.

57. Lipomatous hypertrophy of the tricuspid annulus (arrow) may also occur and may simulate a cardiac tumor. This patient also has a pericardial effusion (*). 2, LV; 3, RA.

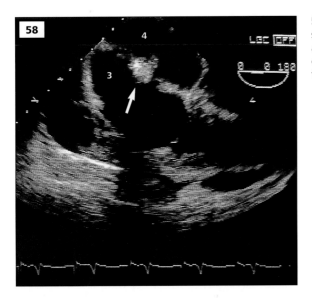

58. Following cardiac transplantation, the thickened suture site (arrow) where the donor heart was anastomosed to the native right atrium may simulate a cardiac mass, as demonstrated in this transesophageal transverse plane four-chamber view. 3, RA; 4, LA.

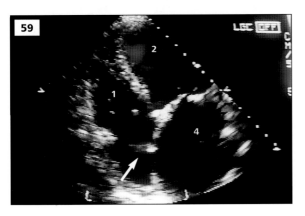

59. A patent foramen ovale is a persistence of the fetal communication from right to left atrium due to failure of fusion of the septum secundum to septum primum. This lack of fusion may allow a flap-like membrane to lift off, which facilitates inter-atrial shunting, predominantly left to right. A probe-patent foramen ovale is present in 28% of autopsied hearts and is seen in 10% of transesophageal studies; it may be an important cause of paradoxical embolus. A color jet across the interatrial septum, consistent with a patent foramen ovale, is seen on this apical four-chamber transthoracic study (arrow). 1, RV; 2, LV; 4, LA.

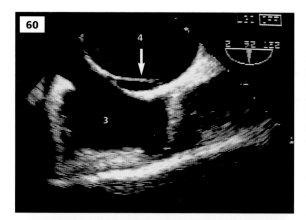

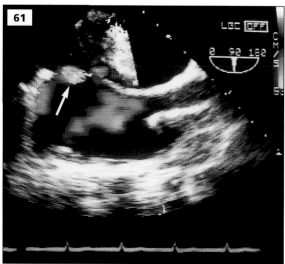

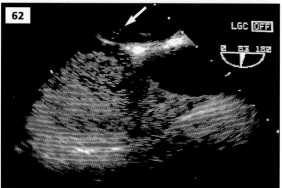

60–62. This longitudinal transesophageal image clearly demonstrates the flap-like membrane of the foramen ovale (**60**) (arrow) which lifts off and, in this instance, allows a small left to right shunt as seen on the color map (arrow) (**61**). This patient had severe mitral regurgitation with elevated left atrial pressure. A few microbubbles are visible in the left atrium following their passage through a patent foramen ovale (arrow) (**62**). 3, RA; 4, LA.

Ventricles

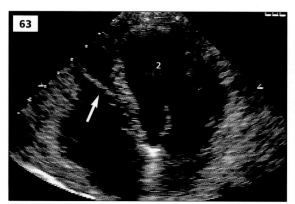

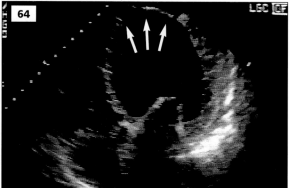

63. The moderator band is a prominent muscular trabeculation or ridge found in the right ventricle of most normal individuals. Echocardiographically, it is best imaged in the apical four-chamber view. The moderator band appears as a dense band (arrow) extending from the lower interventricular septum across the right ventricular cavity to the base of the anterior papillary muscle. 2, LV.

64. Left ventricular false tendons or aberrant bands are fibrous structures that traverse the left ventricular cavity and are considered anatomic variants. It is probable that they are found towards the apex in almost every individual. Unlike true chordae tendineae, which originate from papillary muscles and insert onto valve leaflets, false tendons run from free wall to free wall, from free wall to ventricular septum, or from papillary muscle to ventricular septum. Echocardiographically, false tendons appear as linear, echo-dense structures that course through the ventricular cavity, seen here in a medial–lateral direction.

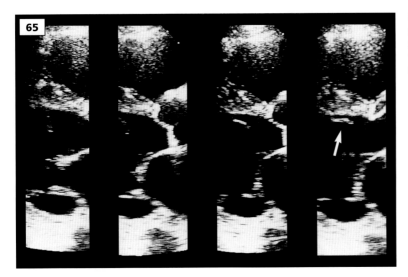

65. Very occasionally these tendons may rupture, usually following a myocardial infarction. In this example the motion of a ruptured tendon is seen (arrow).

Reverberation artifacts and ghosting

Reverberations are secondary reflections that occur along the path of a sound pulse, delaying the return of the signal to the transducer and resulting in the target being displayed multiple times at successively greater depths.

Two characteristic patterns may occur as a result of the internal reverberation of echoes:

- *The sound pulse is reflected back to the transducer from the target and strikes the transducer. It may then be reflected back to the target and then to the transducer a second time. This produces a second echo that is twice the distance of the first echo from the transducer.*
- *If a target is composed of several highly reflective surfaces, the sound pulse may be reflected back and forth several times by the interfaces before returning to the transducer. This produces a series of echoes behind the target.*

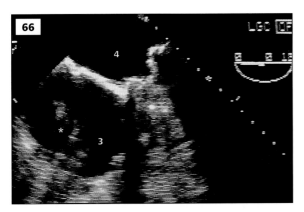

66. In this transverse transesophageal view reverberations from a metal mitral prosthesis (*) produce a 'ghost' image in the right atrium, which may simulate an intracardiac mass. Reverberations – as in this case between the target and transducer – are displayed at twice the distance of the primary target from the transducer and the amplitude of motion of the ghost will be twice that of the original target. 3, RA; 4, LA.

Man-made objects in the heart

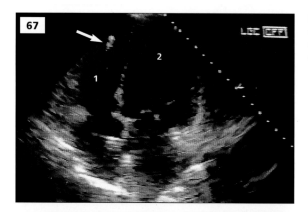

67. Transvenous catheters, including pacing wires, are echo-reflective and may be visualized by echocardiography. In this image the bright tip of a ventricular pacing wire can be seen in the right ventricle. 1, RV; 2, LV.

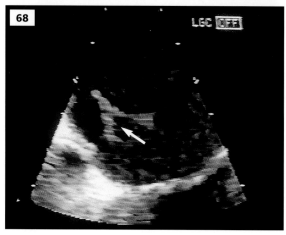

68. Although catheter echos do not in themselves imply an abnormality, transvenous catheters may be the focus for infection and therefore their course should be carefully examined for abnormal echos. In this example, a mobile mass consistent with vegetation (arrow) was seen attached to a left atrial line in a patient with unexplained pyrexia following cardiac transplantation.

Intra-operative echocardiography

Transesophageal echocardiography is being used with increasing frequency to guide and assess cardiac surgery. Imaging may be affected by the use of diathermy; in addition, structures such as the surgeon's finger and intracavitary air produce characteristic appearances.

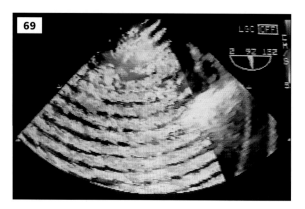

69. Radiofrequency interference from the diathermy produces a 'pinwheel' artifact obscuring both the two-dimensional and color images.

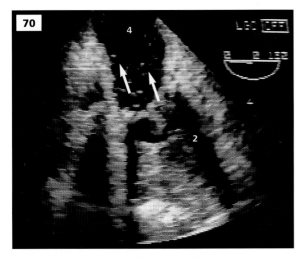

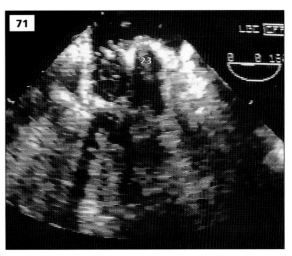

70. Air seen as microbubbles occurs following manual break up of an air pocket (arrows). 2, LV; 4, LA.

71. A surgeon's index finger (23) inserted through the right atrium and displacing the interatrial septum.

Miscellaneous

A large hiatus hernia may impinge on the left atrium and simulate an extracardiac mass. The posterior location and typical presence of swirling stomach contents and air aid in the diagnosis, as can having the patient drink a carbonated beverage during the (transthoracic) examination.

Difficulty in vizualizing the heart on transesophageal echo from the midesophageal or transgastric portion suggests the presence of a hiatus hernia.

The significance of a normal variant frequently relates to the clinical situation and the quality of the images available for interpretation. Minor abnormalities, such as ventricular tendons and vestigial atrial bands, are common and readily recognized; however, the clinical importance of atrial septal aneurysms, patent foramen ovale, and reverberation artifacts needs to be assessed in relation to the patient's status.

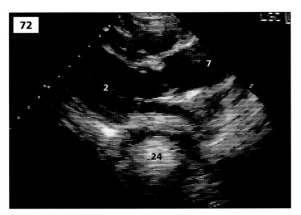

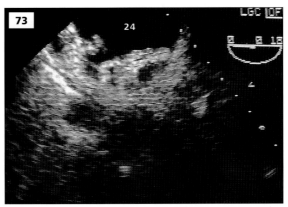

72, 73. A rounded mass is seen posterior to the left atrium on this parasternal long-axis view (**72**). The posterior location and swirling appearance of the contents at transesophageal study (**73**) are in keeping with a large hiatus hernia (24). 2, LV; 7, AO.

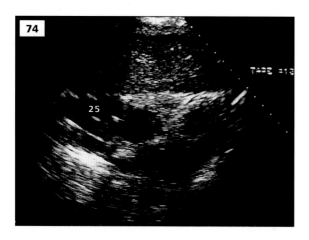

74. Pericardial cyst (25). A benign or Springwater pericardial cyst usually lies across the atrial side of the heart. They are often seen as masses adjacent to the cardiac silhouette or on chest radiograph. They may be difficult to image on echocardiography because of their location but often, as in this case, may be seen by subcostal imaging on deep inspiration.

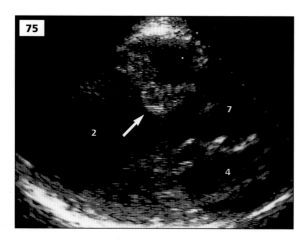

75. In older patients there may be increased angulation between the ventricular septum and aortic root. This increased angle leads to a bulge of muscle below the aortic valve which is pronounced in patients with left ventricular hypertrophy. In this parasternal long-axis view, a bulge is seen below the aortic valve (arrow). This needs to be differentiated from hypertrophic cardiomyopathy and may lead to difficulties. 2, LV; 4, LA; 7, AO.

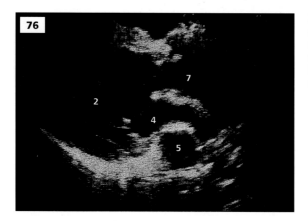

76. If the descending aorta is particularly tortuous it may come to appear to lie within the left atrium. This can be differentiated from membranes within the atrium by turning the transducer through 90° and seeing the longitudinal nature of this structure and the systolic flow within. 2, LV; 4, LA; 5, DAO; 7, AO.

3 RHEUMATIC MITRAL VALVE DISEASE

While the incidence of rheumatic mitral valve disease is declining in western countries, it remains a major health problem in some developing nations. In the West, most patients with rheumatic mitral disease are elderly and have calcified and thickened valves with left atrial enlargement and atrial fibrillation. In developing countries, patients are younger and have thin and pliable valves with a characteristic domed appearance without obvious subvalvar involvement. The early stages of rheumatic involvement are evident as commissural fusion and doming of the mitral valve.

The echocardiographic approach to examining the mitral valve with suspected obstruction is initially to undertake parasternal long- and short-axis views. The long-axis view shows the hooking or doming of the anterior leaflet and the immobility of the posterior leaflet. The thickness of the valve can be measured, as well as any calcification in the valve or annulus. The subvalvar apparatus may be seen in the parasternal long-axis views, though it is best to examine this in apical views. The short-axis view allows direct measurement of the mitral orifice if there is not extensive calcification or a previous valvotomy. The nature of commissural fusion may be examined – an important point in patients considered for conservative surgery or mitral balloon valvotomy.

The mobility of the leaflets and associated left atrial enlargement and thrombus is probably best appreciated in apical views. The presence of coexisting pulmonary hypertension with tricuspid regurgitation can readily be assessed by Doppler interrogation of the tricuspid valve. The mitral orifice area is readily obtained by interrogation using continuous-wave Doppler of the mitral valve from the apex, and allows measurement of the orifice using the pressure half-time method. The correlation between short-axis parasternal measurements of the mitral orifice area by planimetry and pressure half-time Doppler estimations is good, but the latter is more reliable in the presence of calcification and previous surgery. Transesophageal echocardiography allows the examination of the left atrium and appendage for the presence of thrombus and the nature of the valve thickening. Calcification is often better appreciated, and any involvement of the subvalvular apparatus may be determined. Transesophageal echocardiography is a pre-requisite for mitral balloon valvotomy because of the need to exclude atrial thrombus.

Suspect mitral stenosis if:

- *Atrial fibrillation.*
- *Pulmonary edema without impaired left ventricular function.*
- *Transient ischemic attack or stroke.*

	Mitral valve area (cm^2)
Normal	*4–5*
Mild stenosis	*>1.5*
Moderate stenosis	*1.0–1.5*
Severe stenosis	*<1.0*

Mitral balloon valvotomy is possible usually if:

- *Mitral leaflets are not heavily thickened or calcified.*
- *Commissural fusion is symmetric.*
- *There is only mild subvalvular thickening.*
- *There is no left atrial or left atrial appendage thrombus on transesophageal echocardiography.*

Table 1. Causes of mitral valve obstruction
Rheumatic
Congenital commissural fusion parachute valve supravalvar mitral ring Lutembacher's syndrome   (associated with atrial septal defect)
Degenerative mitral annular calcification
Left atrial myxoma
Ball thrombus in left atrium
Cor triatriatum
Mitral annular and leaflet tumors

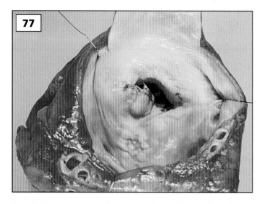

77. Pathologic specimen of the mitral valve. The mitral valve is viewed through the open left atrium. The left atrium is thickened and there is thrombus in the left atrial appendage. The mitral valve is thickened and there is commissural fusion with the formation of a button-hole orifice.

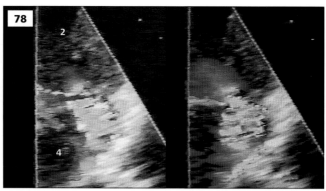

78. Systolic and diastolic frames in an apical four-chamber view. This shows that there is acute mitral regurgitation of no more than mild-to-moderate severity in a young child with acute rheumatic fever. The patient has a Carey–Coombs murmur of mitral regurgitation and at a later date the valve may stenose. The echo features are of commissural fusion and doming of the valve leaflets. 2, LV; 4, LA.

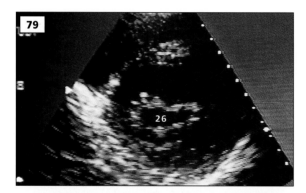

79. Young patient with rheumatic mitral regurgitation. In this short-axis view there is fusion of the commissures (especially the antero-lateral) and a narrowed mitral orifice (26).

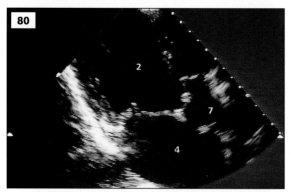

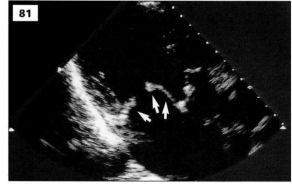

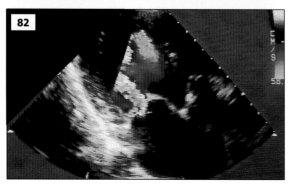

80–82. Apical long-axis view showing the rheumatic mitral valve, left ventricular outflow tract and aortic valve. This is a rather more thickened mitral valve in systole (**80**) which domes in diastole (arrows) (**81**). The edges of the valve are thickened and there is little calcification around the annulus of the mitral valve. Color flow Doppler shows a turbulent jet of increased blood flow velocity through this narrowed orifice (**82**). The left atrium is moderately enlarged. 2, LV; 4, LA; 7, AO.

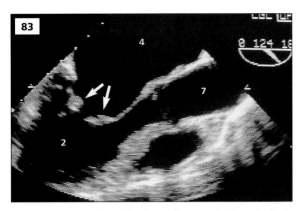

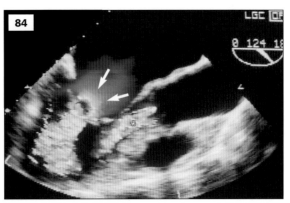

83, 84. Transesophageal echocardiogram in diastole (**83**) and with a color map (**84**). There is mild thickening of a moderately mobile valve. The doming of the valve is well seen (arrows). The left atrium is moderately enlarged.

The color map shows prominent flow convergence (arrows) on the atrial side of the stenotic mitral valve and there is also a jet of aortic regurgitation (*). 2, LV; 4, LA; 7, AO.

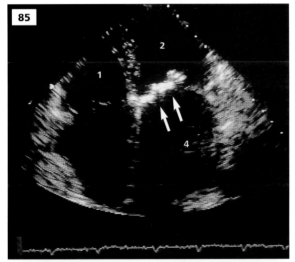

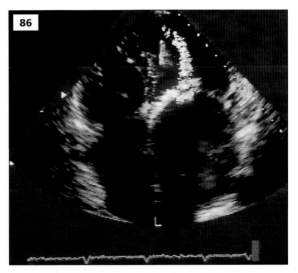

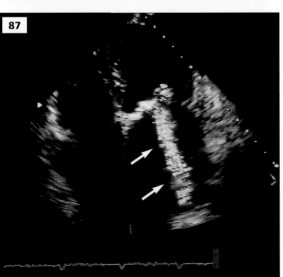

85–87. Apical four-chamber views in a patient with severe long-standing rheumatic mitral stenosis with a very heavily calcified valve, particularly of the anterior leaflet (arrows). In early diastole, the valve is hardly open, but color-flow imaging shows a narrow, non-laminar jet of color Doppler through the valve towards the apex. The left atrium is considerably enlarged. In systole, there is a narrow, non-laminar jet of color Doppler reaching to the back wall of the left atrium (arrows). In mixed mitral valve disease, the length, and even the area of the regurgitant jet by color flow, is not closely related to the severity of mitral regurgitation. 1, RV; 2, LV; 4, LA.

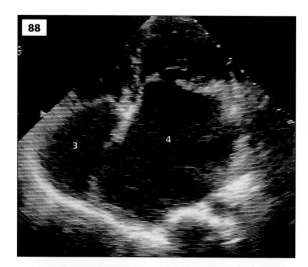

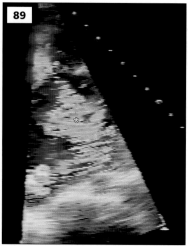

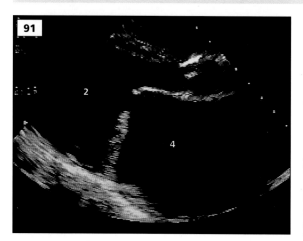

88–90. End-stage of rheumatic mitral valve disease. In this example, there is a huge left atrium with bulging of the inter-atrial septum into the right atrium. There is echo drop-out in the area of the foramen ovale. The mitral valve is calcified and extremely immobile with an orifice area of 1.1 cm² demonstrated by continuous-wave Doppler (see below). The predominant lesion is of mitral regurgitation. The color-flow Doppler shows a jet arising at the center of the mitral orifice and gradually broadening and becoming more mosaic as it reaches the back wall of this huge atrium (*) (**89**). There is a suggestion of laminated thrombus on the posterior aspect of the left atrium. Such thrombus is better examined by transesophageal echocardiography. The transesophageal echocardiogram shows the disorganization and calcification of the valve (**90**). 2, LV; 3, RA; 4, LA.

It may be difficult to assess the severity of mitral regurgitation in patients with long-standing severe rheumatic mitral valve disease. The length and width of regurgitant jets are even more unreliable than usual in the presence of gross left atrial enlargement and a calcified immobile valve.

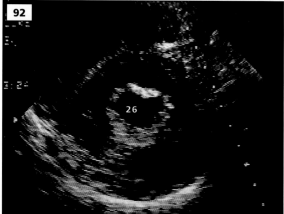

91, 92. Following conservative mitral surgery, such as a closed or open valvotomy, the appearance of the valve is often extremely thickened and immobile. Only in young patients undergoing surgery is there return of anything like the normal movement of the mitral valve. The parasternal long-axis view shows the valve is thickened and immobile (**91**). The short-axis view shows the mitral orifice (26) not to be particularly restricted but with fusion of both commissures and a little calcification around the free edges of the valve (**92**). 2, LV; 4, LA.

Assessment of mitral stenosis is reliable by planimetry in uncalcified valves and by Doppler at slow heart rates. Planimetry is also a more accurate measure than pressure half time by Doppler in the first 2 days after mitral balloon valvotomy. Care must be taken not to cut the leaflet tips obliquely. The planimetered measurements are less reproducible in the presence of an immobile calcified thickened valve, and Doppler is increasingly less reliable as the heart rate rises and the degree of regurgitation rises.

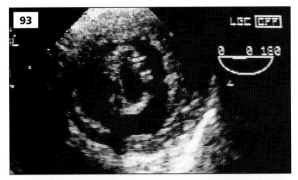

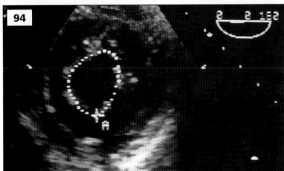

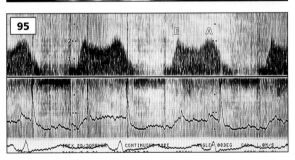

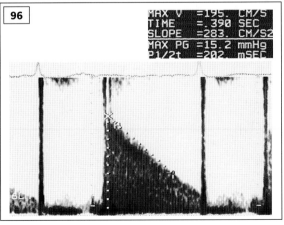

An example of a short-axis view for planimetry is shown in a patient with mild mitral stenosis (**92**) and by transesophageal echocardiography from the transgastric view (**93, 94**). An example of continuous-wave Doppler interrogation of the mitral orifices is shown. This patient is in sinus rhythm (**95**). The slow decline of velocities is seen in early diastole and an atrial peak is seen. The presence of an atrial peak often makes it much more difficult to determine the pressure half-time. In atrial fibrillation, there may be beat-to-beat variation in the pressure half-time (**96**). In addition, there may also be mitral regurgitation – seen as a broad jet away from the transducer. The nature of the mitral regurgitant jet by continuous-wave Doppler has no clear relationship to the severity of regurgitation.

The shape and timing of the mitral stenotic continuous-wave Doppler signal is similar to that in aortic regurgitation. The velocity of the signal is helpful in differentiating these pathologies. The initial velocity in mitral stenosis is always <3 m/s, whereas in aortic regurgitation it is always 3–4 m/s.

93–96. Measurement of the mitral valve orifice area may be made directly by planimetry of short-axis views. This can be performed either transthoracically or by transesophageal short-axis views. Such measurements are reliable, but become less so in the presence of previous surgery or calcification of the valve edges. The alternative method is of Doppler pressure half-time analysis using a continuous-wave probe. The pressure half-time method utilizes the fact that the rate of decline of a mitral pressure gradient is directly proportional to the valve area. In mild stenosis the transvalvular gradient may persist for only a portion of diastole while in severe obstruction the gradient tends to be present throughout the diastole. The pressure half-time provides a quantitative index of the rate of decay of this gradient and was initially introduced as a method of estimating valve area from catheterization data and later was applied to Doppler methods. By definition, the pressure half-time equals the time required for the pressure gradient to fall to one-half of its original value. An empirical formula relating the Doppler half-time to mitral valve area was subsequently provided:
Mitral valve area (cm^2) = 220/pressure half-time (ms).

Complications of Rheumatic Mitral Disease

With increasing severity of rheumatic mitral valve obstruction, the pulmonary artery pressure will rise in response to increasing left atrial pressure and there may be pulmonary hypertension. The subsequent right ventricular pressure overload may lead to tricuspid regurgitation.

The majority of patients with rheumatic mitral valve disease in the West are elderly and have evidence of pulmonary hypertension. There is often gross atrial enlargement and examination for thrombus is imperative.

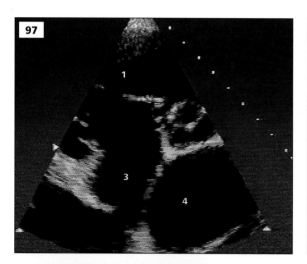

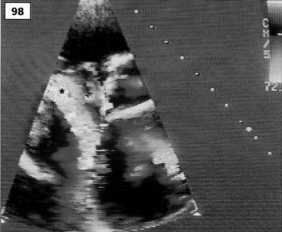

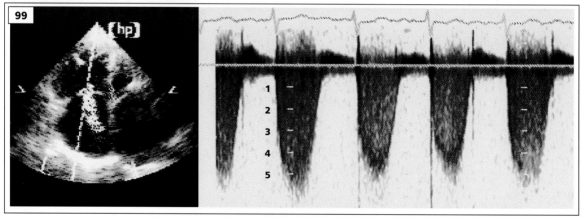

97–99. Parasternal short-axis views showing the right and left atrium and tricuspid valve. The tricuspid valve in this case is structurally normal, but is severely regurgitant due to pulmonary hypertension. A jet of color-flow Doppler is seen arising from the center of the valve and running down the interatrial septum (*) (**98**). Continuous-wave Doppler interrogation of this jet of tricuspid regurgitation is a useful indication of the severity of pulmonary hypertension, which in this case is very severe (**99**). 1, RV; 3, RA; 4, LA.

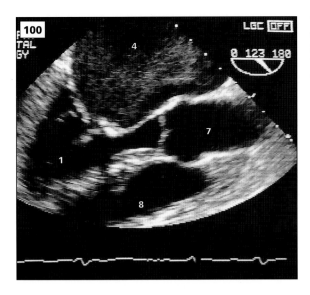

100. Transesophageal echocardiographic demonstration of spontaneous echo contrast in the left atrium is a significant risk factor for the development or presence of thrombus. These findings are seen here in a patient with severe rheumatic mitral stenosis with a huge left atrium. 1, RV; 4, LA; 7, AO; 8, RVOT.

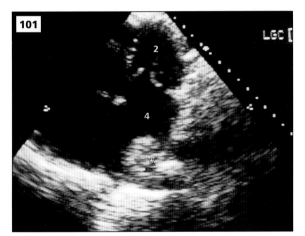

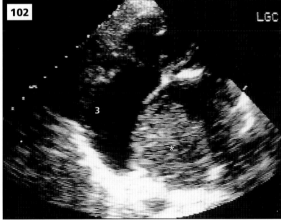

101, 102. Apical four-chamber view showing a huge, rounded homogeneous mass at the back wall of a grossly enlarged left atrium (*). This lies between two pulmonary veins in a patient with mixed mitral valve disease. It can be difficult to differentiate such masses from an atrial myxoma, but the absence of a pedicle and origin away from the interatrial septum, as well as its homogeneity, would suggest this was thrombus. Thrombus classically arises initially within the left atrial appendage and is best seen using transesophageal echocardiography (see **334, 335**). 2, LV; 3, RA; 4, LA.

All patients considered for mitral balloon valvotomy require transesophageal echocardiography to detect atrial thrombus, which is an absolute contradiction to the procedure.

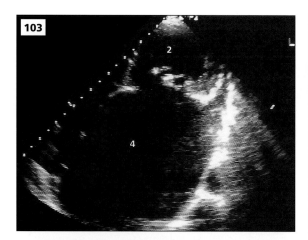

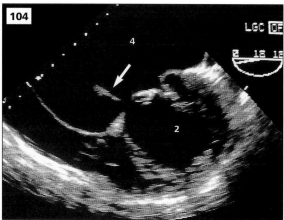

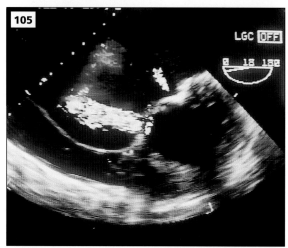

103–105. Complications of mitral balloon valvotomy may be detected by transthoracic and transesophageal echocardiography. In this case there is a torn mitral valve (**103**) with prolapse into the left atrium. This is better seen by transesophageal echo (**104**) (arrow). A color map demonstrates severe mitral regurgitation through the torn portion of valve (**105**). 2, LV; 4, LA.

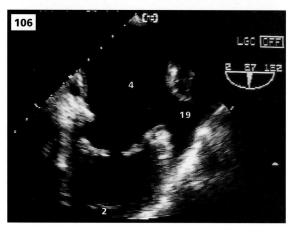

106. Very occasionally, mitral stenosis is not due to rheumatic disease but is of congenital origin. The valve has a thickened diaphragmatic appearance but the physical findings are similar. It is often associated with single papillary muscles, parachute mitral valve, and other forms of left heart atresia, including supra valvar rings, and subvalvar and supra valvar aortic stenosis. Mitral atresia is dealt with in Congenital Heart Disease (pp. 135–152). 2, LV; 4, LA; 19, LAA.

The accuracy of echo Doppler valve area measurements in congenital mitral stenosis is similar to that in rheumatic mitral stenosis.

4 NON-RHEUMATIC MITRAL VALVE DISEASE

The vast majority of cases of mitral regurgitation in the West are due to non-rheumatic or 'floppy' mitral valve disease. This is a degenerative form of connective tissue disorder which, in its mildest form, affects the mitral valve by producing redundancy and floppiness. Subsequently, this valve becomes significantly regurgitant in a small proportion of patients. The use of echocardiography has been essential in the diagnosis and management of such patients. In its simplest form it will show prolapse of the posterior leaflet of the mitral valve associated clinically with a typical click and late systolic murmur of mitral valve prolapse. In its most severe forms there may be prolapse of both leaflets and the complications of this condition, such as ruptured chordae tendineae and mitral valvular dilatation.

Non-rheumatic causes of mitral regurgitation are shown in *Table 2*, while Doppler assessment of the severity of mitral regurgitation is shown in *Table 3*.

Table 2.
Non-rheumatic causes of mitral regurgitation

Congenital
cleft leaflet
double orifice mitral valve
endocardial cushion
  defects
	Ischemic
	papillary muscle
	  dysfunction
	ruptured papillary
	  muscle
	annular dilatation

Mitral valve prolapse floppy valve degenerative collagen vascular disorders Marfan's Ehlers–Danlos osteogenesis imperfecta	**Infective** endocarditis
	Mitral annular calcification
Functional annular dilatation ischemic cardiomyopathy	**Rare** amyloid systemic lupus erythematosus endomyocardial fibrosis

Table 3.
Doppler assessment of the severity of mitral regurgitation

Qualititative	• Continuous wave Doppler signal strength (relative to inflow signal amplitude) *large regurgitant volumes usually produce strong harsh signals* • Systolic profile of the continuous wave Doppler recordings *early systolic fall in jet velocity in severe regurgitation with "V" waves* • Increase in mitral inflow velocity in the absence of mitral stenosis *peak velocity >2 m/s implies severe regurgitation*
Semi-quantitative	• Assessment of color Doppler jet length and area compared to size of left atrium *remember color Doppler flow mapping displays velocity information not volume data wall jets may be underestimated (Coanda effect)* • Decreased or reversed pulmonary venous systolic flow in severe mitral regurgitation (best assessed by transesophageal echocardiography)
Quantitative (not routine clinical use)	**1. Proximal isovelocity surface area (PISA) calculations** • Regurgitant flow rate = $2\pi r^2 \times$ aliasing velocity • Regurgitant orifice area = $\dfrac{\text{Regurgitant flow rate}}{\text{Regurgitant velocity}}$ • Regurgitant volume = Regurgitant orifice area $\times$ Regurgitant VTI **2. Spectral Doppler calculations** • Regurgitant fraction = $\dfrac{(\text{mitral orifice area} \times \text{mitral VTI}) \ (\text{LVOT area} \times \text{LVOT VTI})}{(\text{mitral orifice area} \times \text{mitral VTI})}$ VTI = velocity time integral LVOT = left ventricular outflow tract

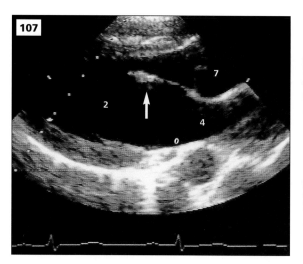

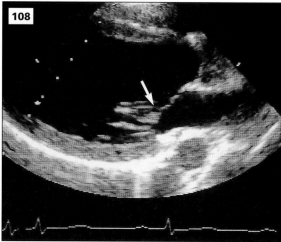

107, 108. Parasternal long-axis views in diastole (**107**) and systole (**108**) showing a redundant myxomatous mitral valve (arrows) without prolapse. 2, LV; 4, LA; 7, AO.

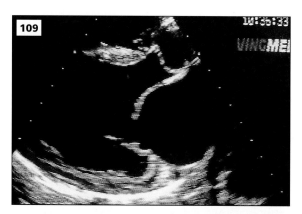

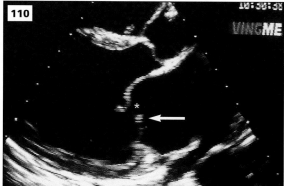

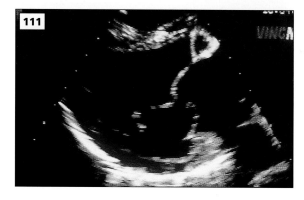

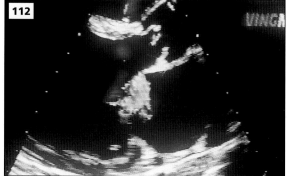

109–112. Sequence of echocardiograms showing prolapse of the posterior leaflet of the mitral valve. In diastole it can be seen there is slight enlargement of the left atrium with normal left ventricular function. As the valve closes, there is failure of coaptation (*) and prolapse of the posterior leaflet (arrow). Color flow Doppler shows that there is a central jet of mitral regurgitation in the area of failure of coaptation.

Mitral valve prolapse occurs in 5% of the population. There is a tendency to overdiagnose mitral valve prolapse due to the fact that the mitral annulus is saddle-shaped. Mitral leaflets which appear normal on a parasternal long-axis view may appear to bow back into the left atrium on an apical four-chamber view. The following are strict criteria for the diagnosis of mitral valve prolapse:

- *Movement of any part of the anterior or posterior leaflet behind the plane of the annulus in a parasternal long-axis view.*
- *Movement of the point of apposition behind the plane of the annulus in the apical four-chamber view.*

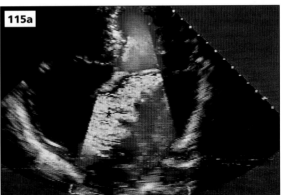

113. Short-axis imaging of the mitral valve in mitral valve prolapse with redundancy of the leaflets in this case of severe mitral prolapse in a patient with Marfan's syndrome. There is a scalloped appearance of both the anterior and posterior leaflets.

If there is predominantly prolapse of one leaflet, the mitral regurgitant jet is eccentric and directed away from that leaflet.

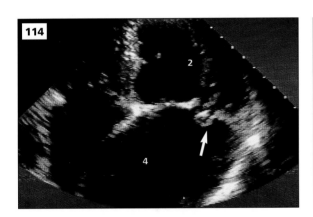

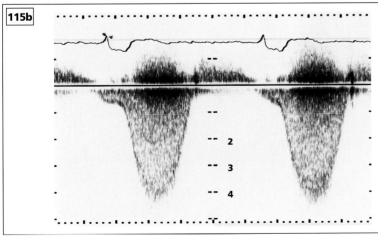

114, 115. The apical four-chamber view is probably the most sensitive and specific view for examining mitral valve prolapse. In this example there is localized prolapse of the posterior leaflet of the mitral valve (**114**, arrow). There is a jet of color flow seen to extend along the anterior leaflet of the mitral valve and along the interatrial septum (**115a**, *). Continuous-wave Doppler will demonstrate a broad jet from the left ventricle to the left atrium. The nature of the jet does not bear a strong relationship with the severity of mitral regurgitation (**115b**). 2, LV; 4, LA.

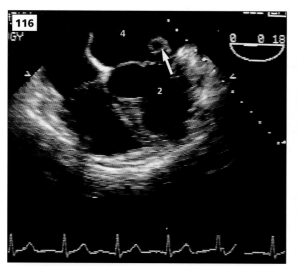

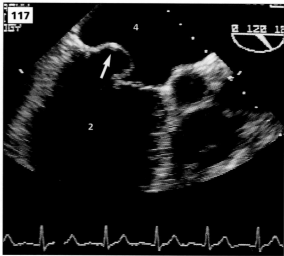

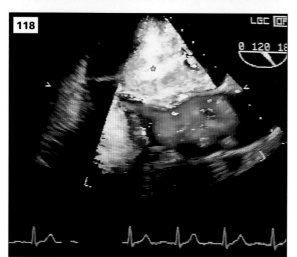

116–118. Transesophageal echocardiographic imaging of the mitral valve in the intra-operative setting is often of particular help in examining the degree and site of mitral prolapse. In this example there is classic posterior leaflet prolapse. In diastole the valve may look relatively normal, but in early systole there is prolapse of the posterior leaflet and this becomes aneurysmal towards the end of systole (seen at 0° and 120°) (arrows). There is an extensive jet of mitral regurgitation seen by color-flow map (*). 2, LV; 4, LA.

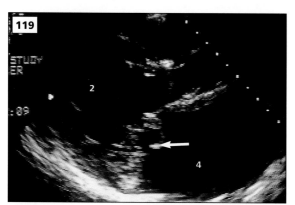

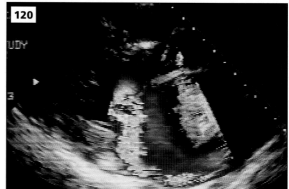

119, 120. While the most common form of mitral prolapse involves the posterior leaflet and this is the most straightforward for operative repair, the anterior leaflet, or both leaflets may be involved. In this example – seen in the parasternal long-axis view – there is calcification or thickening of the posterior mitral valve and annulus, but there is prolapse with ruptured chordae of the anterior leaflet (arrow). This produces an aneurysmal appearance and is the site of mitral regurgitation seen by color-flow imaging. 2, LV; 4, LA.

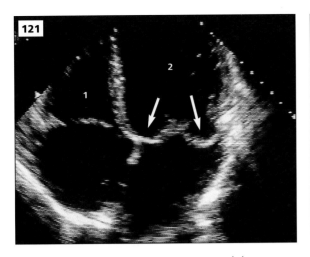

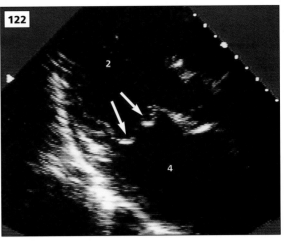

121, 122. Apical long-axis images may reveal the prolapse of both leaflets. In diastole, the mitral valve looks essentially normal, but in systole there is obvious prolapse behind the closure line of both anterior and posterior leaflets as seen in a mild (**121**) and severe (**122**) example (arrows). 1, RV; 2, LV; 4, LA.

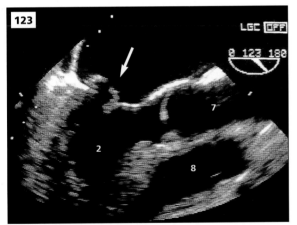

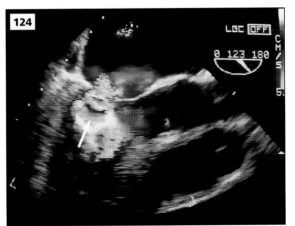

123, 124. Transesophageal echocardiography in prolapse of both leaflets of the mitral valve. The leaflet tissue is greatly redundant and scalloped, with an aneurysmal appearance being seen in the left atrium (arrow). The color map shows a large flow convergent region on the ventricular side of the regurgitant valve. The size of the flow convergent region is considered a parameter of severity of mitral regurgitation (arrow). 2, LV; 7, AO; 8, RVOT.

In degenerative mitral valve disease with prolapse of a mitral valve leaflet, ruptured chordae tendinae may appear on transesophageal imaging as mobile bright masses attached to the leaflet. It is important to be aware of this appearance to ensure that these structures are not misinterpreted as vegetations.

Mitral regurgitant jets usually appear larger in area on transesophageal echo compared with transthoracic scanning. This must be taken into account when grading the severity of mitral regurgitation.

Despite many recent technical advances, echocardiography remains unreliable in the assessment of mitral regurgitation. Imaging may reveal the anatomic substrate for mitral regurgitation with leaflet prolapse and annular dilatation, but assesment of volume loading of the left ventricle and Doppler jets does not reliably quantify the regurgitant fraction. Jets impinging on a wall are particularly difficult to quantify as they cannot expand and produce smaller color flow areas than a similar regurgitant volume directed centrally (Coanda effect).

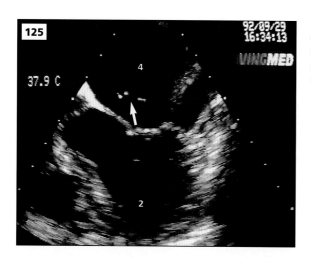

125. Ruptured chordae are often readily seen by transesophageal echocardiography because of its superior imaging in comparison with transthoracic imaging. In this example a ruptured chord is seen moving within the left atrium in systole (arrow). 2, LV; 4, LA.

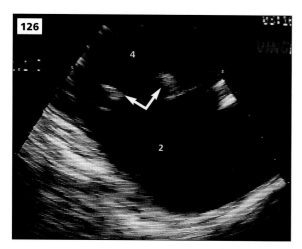

126. In association with non-rheumatic mitral regurgitation the valve anterior leaflet may have a deep cleft within it. This is often the site of regurgitation. It may be associated with atrial septal defect, particularly of the atrioventricular septal defect type. In this example the anterior leaflet of the mitral valve looks relatively normal in diastole, but in systole a deep cleft is seen occupying one half of the anterior leaflet. 2, LV; 4, LA.

127, 128. Ventricular dilatation, whether due to cardiomyopathy or ischemia, may produce incomplete mitral valve closure and functional mitral regurgitation. This is due to the apical displacement of the papillary muscles, which puts tension on the leaflets and displaces their coaptation apically. The role of mitral annular dilatation in the etiology of functional mitral regurgitation is less certain. In Figure **127**, the apical displacement of the papillary muscles in this very dilated left ventricle 'tents' the mitral leaflets, with resultant incomplete closure on this apical four-chamber view. The corresponding color-flow image (**128**) demonstrates the central regurgitant jet (*). 2, LV; 4, LA.

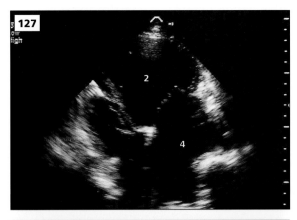

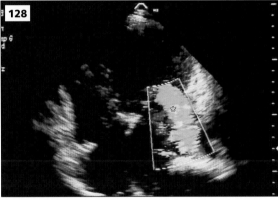

129. Mitral annular calcification is a degenerative disorder seen in elderly people. Calcification of the posterior mitral annulus occurs far more frequently than calcification of the anterior annulus. It may be associated with mitral regurgitation, conduction defects, and endocarditis. It may also pose difficulties if mitral valve surgery is contemplated. In this example the parasternal short-axis view shows a dense rim of calcium extending from the medial to lateral posterior margins of the annulus (*).

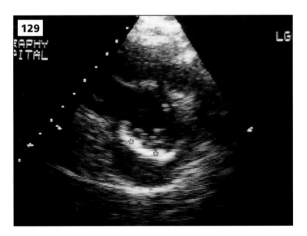

Mitral Valve Surgery

Mitral valve repair of non-rheumatic mitral regurgitation is now the treatment of choice. It is considered that retention of the subvalvular structures preserves left ventricular function better than following mitral prosthetic insertion with excision of the papillary muscles. In addition, if the patient is in sinus rhythm, life-long anticoagulation is not required. Mitral repair consists of inserting a flexible or rigid annuloplasty ring onto the atrial aspect of the mitral valve. This reduces the annular dimension and allows coaptation of the leaflets. It is often necessary to resect and plicate the redundant leaflet tissue.

Surgery should be performed in severe mitral regurgitation before the onset of irreversible left ventricular dysfunction. In acute mitral regurgitation the left ventricle is hyperdynamic and not dilated. In chronic mitral regurgitation the left ventricle dilates and eventually irreversible dysfunction occurs. Where possible, mitral valve repair is the procedure of choice. Repair of posterior leaflet prolapse is relatively straightforward and involves leaflet resection and the insertion of an annuloplasty ring. Repair of anterior leaflet prolapse is more difficult; anterior leaflet resection is not feasible but depending on the degree of prolapse, chordal transfer may be undertaken.

Intra-operative transesophageal echocardiography allows appropriate planning of the mitral repair, determining the presence and severity of chordal rupture and leaflet prolapse (particularly the anterior, which is more difficult to repair). Also, the final outcome may be assessed by determining the presence and severity of regurgitation after the termination of cardiopulmonary bypass and before chest closure. Moderate residual regurgitation may be an indication for a further attempt at repair or a replacement.

The pre-operative echo should assess:

- *Site and degree of prolapse of each leaflet.*
- *Severity of mitral regurgitation.*
- *Annular calcification.*
- *Left ventricular function.*

The post-operative echo should assess:

- *Residual leaflet prolapse.*
- *Degree of mitral regurgitation.*
- *'Seating' of the annuloplasty ring.*
- *Evidence of mitral stenosis.*
- *Evidence of left ventricular outflow tract obstruction.*
- *Left ventricular function.*

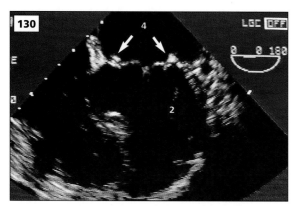

130. Transesophageal echocardiogram immediately postoperatively, showing (arrows) the annuloplasty ring as bright structures. The valve which was previously redundant has been plicated with a posterior resection. The posterior leaflet has a characteristic 'stubby' appearance following this. 2, LV; 4, LA.

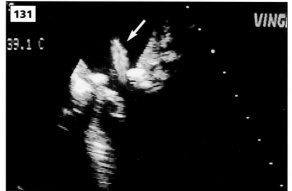

131. Following a mitral valve repair it may be difficult to define the detail of the valve. On this transesophageal echocardiogram the bright echos of the annuloplasty ring are seen, but there is mild residual regurgitation, as seen by color-flow mapping (arrow).

5 MITRAL VALVE REPLACEMENT

The variety of types of mitral valve replacements available – both biological and mechanical – are listed in *Table 4*.

Biological Valves

The Doppler parameters of biological mitral valve replacements are listed in *Table 5*.

Echocardiography of biological valves shows the porcine valve and the mounting stent. The porcine valve is made up of two pig aortic valves and appears very similar to a normally functioning aortic valve. The cusps are thin and mobile, and it is not for many years that they become thickened and initially stenotic. Stenosis usually precedes fracture of a cusp; the subsequent regurgitation is often acute and severe.

Full assessment of prosthetic valve dysfunction requires both transthoracic and transesophageal studies due to masking by the prosthesis and reverberation artifact.

Table 4. Mitral valve replacements

Biological

Homograft (stented)
cadaveric aortic and pulmonary valves

Xenograft
porcine aortic valve:
• Carpentier–Edwards
• Hancock
bovine pericardium: Ionescu–Shiley

Mechanical

Ball and cage: Starr–Edwards

Single tilting disc:
• Björk–Shiley
• Hall–Medtronics
• Lillehei Kaster
• Omniscience

Bileaflet:
• St Jude Medical
• Carbomedics
• Duromedics

Table 5. Doppler parameters in biological mitral bioprostheses

	Peak velocity (m/s)	Peak gradient (mmHg)	Mean gradient (mmHg)	Mitral valve area (cm^2)
Carpentier–Edwards (porcine valve)	1.8 ± 0.2	12.5 ± 3.6	6.5 ± 2.1	2.5 ± 0.7
Hancock (porcine valve)	1.5 ± 0.3	9.7 ± 3.2	4.3 ± 2.1	1.6 ± 0.4
Ionescu–Shiley (pericardial valve)	1.5 ± 0.3	8.5 ± 2.9	3.3 ± 1.2	2.4 ± 0.8

All valvular prostheses show some degree of both stenosis and regurgitation.

Examination of a valve prosthesis should address the following questions:

- *Is the prosthesis well-seated?*
- *Is mobility of discs, leaflets, and/or ball normal?*
- *Are any abnormal masses or cavities present (thrombus, vegetations, abscess)?*
- *Is the prosthesis stenosed?*
- *Is there pathologic regurgitation?*

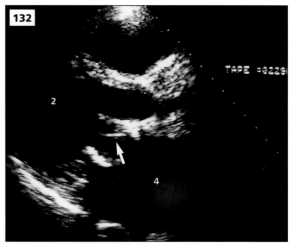

132. Echocardiogram of a porcine xenograft showing a stent and thin cusps (arrow). 2, LV; 4, LA.

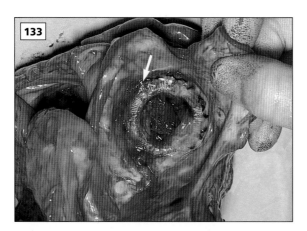

133. Autopsy specimen of a failed mitral xenograft – this is of the Hancock-type and there is a pannus of thrombus and inflammatory tissue growing across the atrial aspect of the implanted valve. The stent (arrowed) and the sewing ring can be seen.

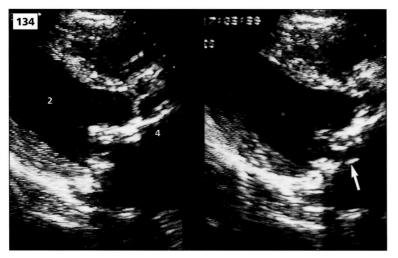

134. Diastolic and systolic frames showing a heavily thickened and immobile valve with a significant increase in blood flow velocity. This may be measured directly with Doppler and, in this case, led to a mitral valve orifice area of 1.1 cm^2. The valve also prolapses in systole but this was not accompanied by severe mitral regurgitation (arrow). 2, LV; 4, LA.

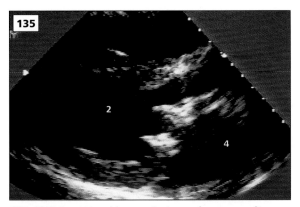

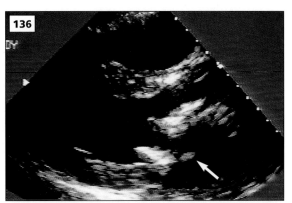

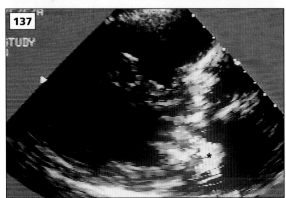

135–137. Parasternal long-axis views of a xenograft mitral valve which has failed some 7 years after implantation. In diastole (**135**), the valve looks thin and the mounting stent normally placed. However, in systole (**136**), there is prolapse of one of the valve leaflets, which is seen clearly in the left atrium (arrow). The forward Doppler flow across this valve is of normal velocity, but in systole there is a broad jet of mitral regurgitation (mosaic of color flow) (*) into the enlarged left atrium (**137**). 2, LV; 4, LA.

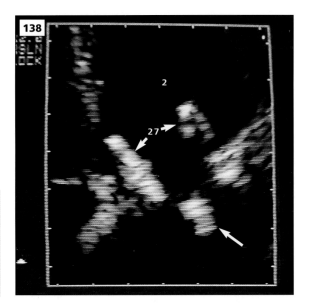

138. The prolapse of the thickened and calcified mitral xenograft cusp is best seen in the apical long-axis view. The magnified view shows the valve to be very thickened, particularly affecting one cusp, which has exaggerated movement in diastole with thickening of its tip and prolapse in systole (arrow). Two stents (27) of the prosthesis are also readily identified. 2, LV; 27, Stent.

Avoid continuous use of color Doppler flow mapping when imaging as it will obscure morphologic detail. Two-dimensional imaging should be performed prior to subsequent color Doppler mapping.

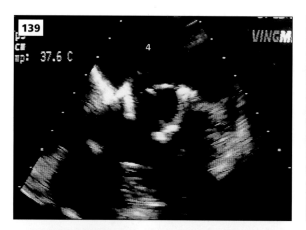

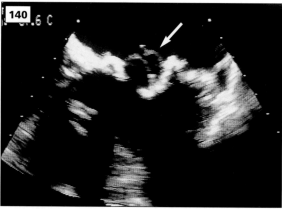

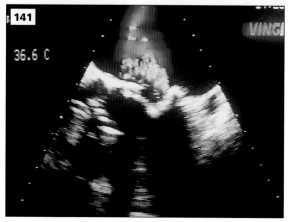

139–141. Transesophageal echocardiography may demonstrate prolapse of xenograft cusps, even if they are not thickened. The valve stents are clearly seen and in early systole the valve appears to be thin and approximates normally (**139**). However, as systole progresses, there is prolapse that particularly affects one cusp (arrow) (**140**). The color map confirms the site of regurgitation (**141**). 4, LA.

In normal biological valves the cusps are approximately 1 mm in diameter and >3 mm is considered abnormal. Biological valve replacements have a very variable rate of deterioration that influences echo assessment. A valve should not have thickened and calcified in the first few years after implantation, but unusually this may be seen, while others appear thin after a decade or more. The development of leaflet prolapse and even mild regurgitation is often the prelude to the onset of increasing severity of regurgitation. Usually, the presence of vegetations is readily apparent, but in old and degenerate valves, thickening and cusp vibration may simulate masses.

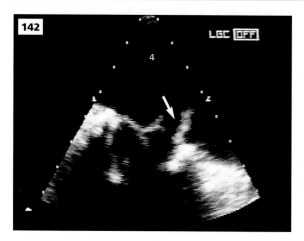

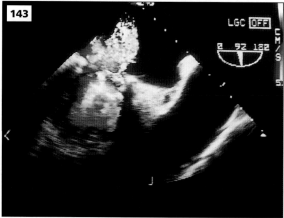

142, 143. Transesophageal echocardiography demonstrating prolapse of both xenograft cusps in a very thickened mitral valve replacement (arrow). There is extensive mitral regurgitation by color map. 4, LA.

Mechanical Valves

The Doppler parameters of mechanical mitral valve replacements are listed in *Table 6*.

Table 6.
Doppler parameters in mechanical mitral prostheses

	Peak velocity (m/s)	Peak gradient (mmHg)	Mean gradient (mmHg)	Mitral valve area (cm^2)
Starr–Edwards	1.9 ± 0.4	14.6 ± 5.5	4.6 ± 2.4	2.0 ± 0.5
St Jude Medical	1.6 ± 0.3	10.0 ± 3.6	3.5 ± 1.3	3.3 ± 0.6
Björk–Shiley	1.6 ± 0.3	10.7 ± 2.7	2.9 ± 1.6	2.2 ± 0.6

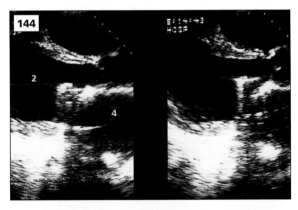

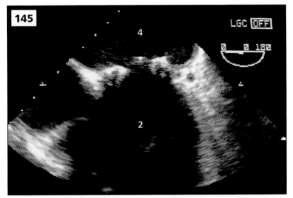

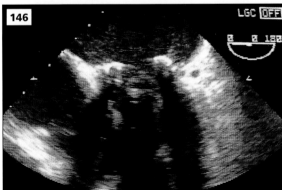

144–147. Transthoracic echocardiographic long-axis images of a normally functioning Starr–Edwards mitral valve replacement (**144**). Because of echo reverberation within the ball and metal frame, it is often difficult to image the valve itself and surrounding structures, especially the left atrium. However, one can appreciate the movement of the ball within the cage. Transesophageal echocardiography is the method of choice for studying the left atrium. In this example, systolic (**145**) and diastolic (**146**) frames are shown and the ball moves normally within the frame. The left atrium is large with spontaneous contrast, but does not contain thrombus. There is masking of the left ventricle by reverberations within the Starr valve. Color flow imaging may show mild mitral regurgitation which is normal for a ball valve. Color mapping of inflow through a Starr prosthesis is distinctive, as the blood has to circumnavigate the ball producing two jets of inflow around the ball valve (**147**). Starr valves are often obstructive, especially the smaller sizes, with orifice areas in the range of 1.4–1.8 cm^2. 2, LV; 4, LA.

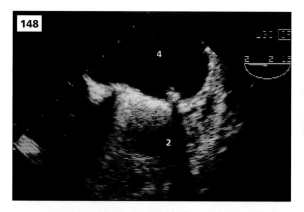

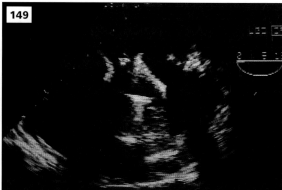

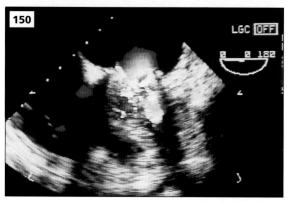

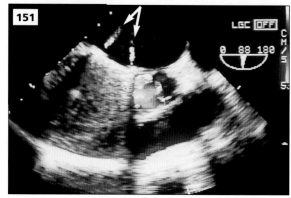

148–151. Normal functioning single disc (Omniscience) mitral valve replacement in systole (**148**) and diastole (**149**) by transesophageal echocardiography. As with other mechanical valves, there is a good deal of masking of the ventricular cavity behind the valve. In diastole, one major inflow jet is visible on color mapping (**150**). In systole, color-flow imaging shows two insignificant jets of mitral regurgitation as the valve closes (**151**, arrows); jets such as these are normal for this type of valve. 2, LV; 4, LA.

- *Transesophageal echo has improved the morphologic assessment of valvular prosthesis because of higher transducer frequency and a superior acoustic window. It is superior to transthoracic imaging for the assessment of mobility of prosthetic discs or leaflets and for the detection of thrombus; it also has greater sensitivity for the detection of vegetation.*

- *Transesophageal echo also permits mapping of the left atrium for prosthetic mitral regurgitation as reverberation artifacts occur on the ventricular side of the prosthesis, unlike in transthoracic imaging in which the left atrium is obscured by reverberations.*

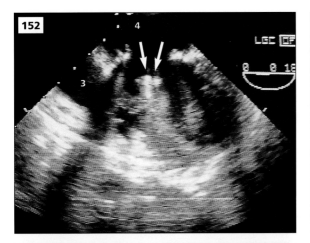

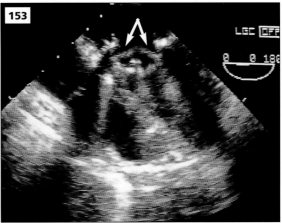

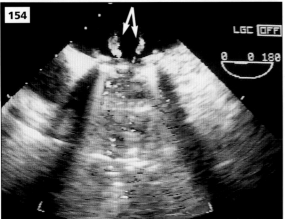

152–154. Transesophageal echocardiography of a normally functioning bileaflet St Jude mitral valve replacement. This shows in diastole (**152**), the two discs opening parallel to flow and forming two parallel lines (arrows). In systole, the two discs close to form an inverted 'V' (**153**) (arrows). Color-flow mapping in systole demonstrates two distinct jets of minimal regurgitation; up to four jets are normal for this type of valve (**154**) (arrows). 3, RA; 4, LA.

- *Normal transvalvular prosthetic regurgitation results from the design of the prosthesis and includes closure volumes due to closure of the occluding device and to leakage backflow, which occurs once the valve is closed fully.*
- *Closure volumes occur with all mechanical valves and approximately 10% of bioprosthetic valves.*
- *Leakage backflow occurs with mechanical valves, except for the Starr–Edwards ball-in-cage because the ball fits snugly in the cage.*
- *The typical patterns of normal transvalvular prosthetic regurgitation are detected by transesophageal echo.*

Failed mechanical mitral replacements

Potential prosthetic valve problems include thrombosis, endocarditis (see Endocarditis, p. 79), paravalvular leak and dehiscence.

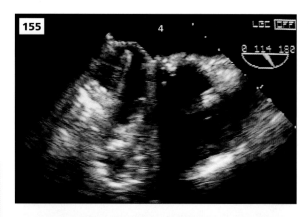

The motion of the valve leaflets of any type of replacement is difficult to visualize. However, when valve movement is restricted by thrombus or infection this is readily seen and the increase in blood velocity simulating mitral stenosis demonstrated by Doppler. Although pressure half-time is not a reliable guide to orifice area in normally functioning mitral prostheses – as it reflects non-prosthetic factors such as left ventricular diastolic behavior more closely – a pressure half-time of >200 ms suggests obstruction, especially if the peak velocity is >2.5 ms.

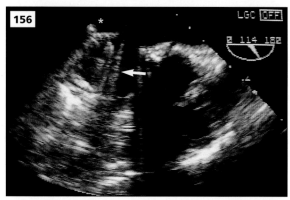

- *It may be difficult to classify tiny mobile structures in the vicinity of prosthetic valves, as detected by transesophageal imaging. These may represent pathology, but may simply be loose suture ends. Interpretation, therefore, must always be made in the clinical context.*

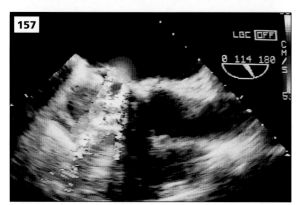

155–157. Systolic (**155**) and diastolic (**156**) frames of an acutely occluded St Jude bileaflet mitral valve replacement. Transesophageal echocardiography was performed due to difficulty in weaning the patient off cardiopulmonary bypass following mitral and aortic valve replacements. In systole, the mitral valve replacement appears normal, but in diastole only one disc opens (arrow) and the other remains stuck in a closed position (*). Color-flow mapping demonstrates an eccentric turbulent jet through the open leaflet (**157**). A piece of chord was found to be obstructing the mitral disc. Following removal of the piece of chord the mitral valve replacement functioned normally. 4, LA.

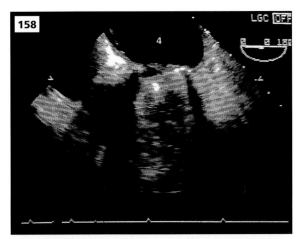

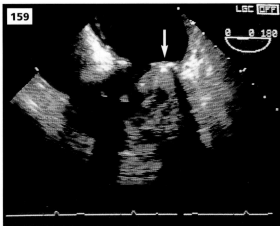

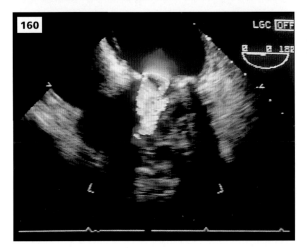

158–160. Thrombotic occlusion of a bileaflet Carbomedics mitral valve replacement. In comparison with (**155**), both discs appear thickened in systole (**158**), while in diastole (**159**) one disc remains stuck in a closed position (arrow). Color-flow imaging demonstrates an eccentric jet through the open disc, with a large area of flow convergence (**160**). At surgery, laminated thrombus was present on both atrial and ventricular aspects of the discs. 4, LA.

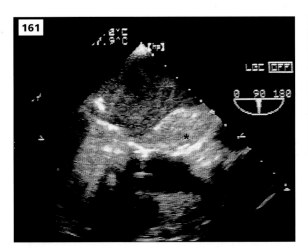

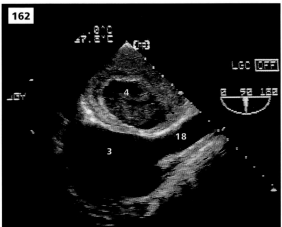

161, 162. Thrombosed Starr–Edwards mitral prosthesis. Transesophageal longitudinal views show thrombus obscuring the ball prosthesis (**161**) with marked spontaneous contrast and a huge laminated thrombus along the left atrial wall (*). The longitudinal bi-atrial view (**162**) shows thrombus filling the left atrium. 3, RA; 4, LA; 18, SVC.

Valve replacements containing metal and carbon elements result in artifacts that may mask features suggestive of malfunction. In addition, one or more short jets of color Doppler may be seen in normal functioning valves. A dehisced valve may rock on its mounting and such disruption may be visualized, especially by transesophageal echocardiography. However, current surgical practice attempts to preserve the subvalvular apparatus to reduce left ventricular impairment. In this situation the valve may appear quite mobile.

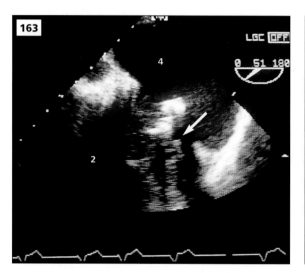

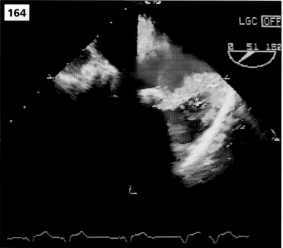

163, 164. Multiplane transesophageal echocardiogram in a Starr–Edwards mitral valve replacement with paravalvular leak. The systolic frame (**163**) shows the site of regurgitation adjacent to the strut (arrow). Color-flow mapping confirms a moderate paravalvular leak at this site (*). Multiplane scanning greatly facilitates detection of such leaks, the longitudinal views being of particular value. 2, LV; 4, LA.

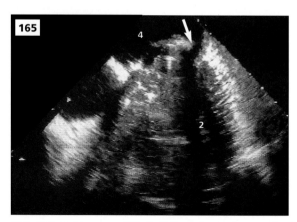

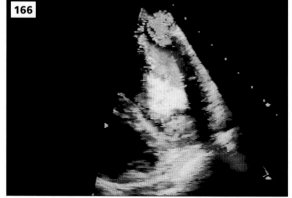

165, 166. Dehiscence of Bjork–Shiley mitral valve prosthesis (arrow) (**165**) with color-flow map confirming severe regurgitation at that site. 2, LV; 4, LA.

6 AORTIC VALVE DISEASE

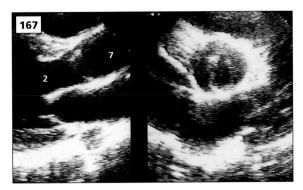

167. Both leaflets of the bicuspid valve are shown to prolapse from their annular insertion. This is not necessarily associated with regurgitation, but is often its precursor. In a short-axis view, the bicuspid nature of the valve can be seen. In this case a distribution of leaflets is of the North–South type, which is a less common form. 2, LV; 7, AO.

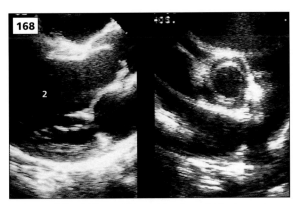

168. A mildly thickened bicuspid valve which domes in systole but is not severely obstructed. The short-axis view (right) shows the valve fully opened with a substantial orifice. The distribution of bicuspid leaflets is of the East–West type which is more common. 2, LV.

Aortic Stenosis

Aortic valve thickening occurs in 20% of the population aged >65 years and is clinically significant in 3% of these and in 10% of those aged >80 years.

Before the development of echocardiography, it was difficult to assess aortic stenosis without cardiac catheterization. Echocardiography will determine the nature of the valve abnormality and whether it is thickened and immobile. The presence of left ventricular hypertrophy and dilatation are important in the assessment of severity. Doppler examination of blood flow velocity will determine the severity of aortic stenosis with a higher degree of reliability. Aortic stenosis can be divided into those of congenital origin, namely bicuspid aortic valves and degenerative three cuspid aortic valve stenosis.

The murmur of aortic stenosis may become soft, or even absent, when left ventricular function is impaired.

Congenital aortic valve disease

Bicuspid aortic valves occur in 1–2% of the population and may be associated with coarctation of the aorta.

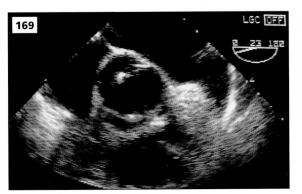

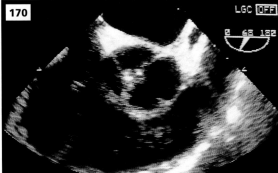

169, 170. Transesophageal echocardiography showing a functionally unobstructed bicuspid aortic valve with fusion of raphae.

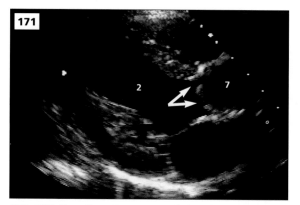

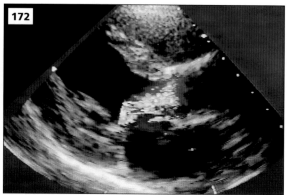

171, 172. Transthoracic parasternal views in a patient with a domed and mildly stenotic bicuspid valve (arrows). In diastole (**171**), the valve prolapses into the left ventricular outflow tract. Both leaflets prolapse equally and there is a jet of aortic regurgitation seen running along the anterior leaflet of the mitral valve (**172**). 2, LV; 7, AO.

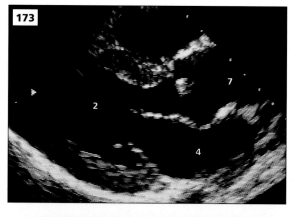

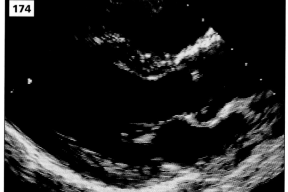

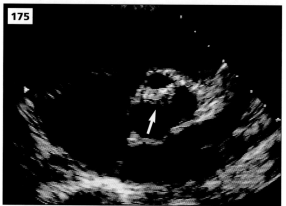

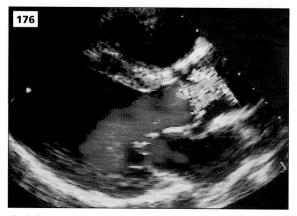

173–176. Increasing severity of aortic stenosis is usually associated with thickening of at least one of the leaflets and left ventricular hypertrophy. There is thickening of the left coronary commissure with fusion of this raphae (arrows). The valve domes in systole and color flow shows a high-velocity forward blood flow. 2, LV; 4, LA; 7, AO.

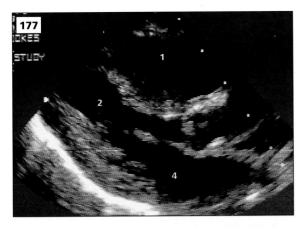

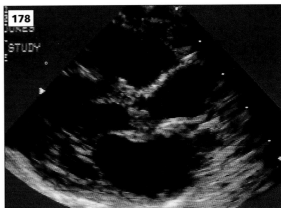

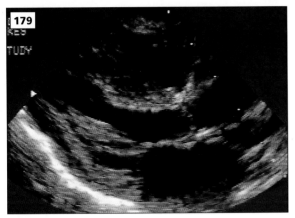

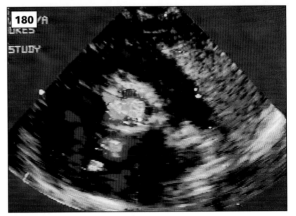

177–180. Aortic stenosis may present in the neonate as the cause of heart failure with low cardiac output. There is a very thickened aortic valve which domes in systole and has redundant tissue. Short-axis views show this to be a unicuspid valve with a narrow jet of central, high-velocity blood flow. It is more common for unicuspid valves to present in early life. For a child of this age, there is significant left ventricular hypertrophy. 1, RV; 2, LV; 4, LA.

- *Bicuspid aortic valve is the most common congenital cardiac anomaly.*

- *Bicuspid valves are clinically important as they may present with significant aortic stenosis in childhood or undergo progressive thickening and eventual obstruction in later years.*

- *Bicuspid valves are frequently incompetent and predispose to endocarditis.*

- *Bicuspid valve may be familial.*

Degenerative aortic valve disease

Assessment of the severity of aortic stenosis by Doppler echocardiography is shown in *Table 7*.

Table 7. Assessment of severity of aortic stenosis by Doppler	
Instantaneous pressure gradient (Bernoulli equation)	$P_1 - P_2 = 4(V_2^2 - V_1^2)$ If $V_1 < 1\text{m/s}$ may be simplified to $\Delta P = 4V_2^2$ P_1 = Peak left ventricular pressure P_2 = Peak aortic pressure V_1 = Peak velocity proximal to obstruction V_2 = Peak stenotic velocity
Velocity ratio	Ratio of peak left ventricular outflow tract velocity to peak aortic velocity (<0.25 implies severe aortic stenosis)
Valve area	**1. Continuity equation** LVOT area × LVOT velocity = Aortic valve area × Peak aortic velocity or Aortic valve area = $\dfrac{\text{LVOT area} \times \text{LVOT velocity}}{\text{Peak aortic velocity}}$ **2. Planimetry** Planimetry of aortic orifice at leaflet tip level by multiplane TEE **3. Cardiac output method** Aortic valve area = $\dfrac{\text{Cardiac output}}{\text{SEP} \times \text{mean post-stenotic velocity}}$ LVOT = left vetricular outflow tract SEP = Systolic ejection period

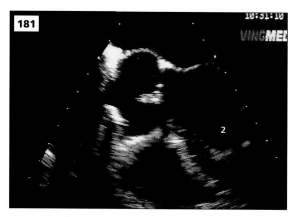
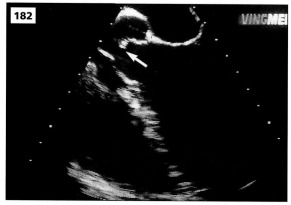

181, 182. With age, the aortic valve thickens and becomes much less mobile. This transesophageal view shows it thickened and domed (arrowed) with some calcium and this is often the source of a murmur. However, the valve opens sufficiently to allow normal flow. 2, LV.

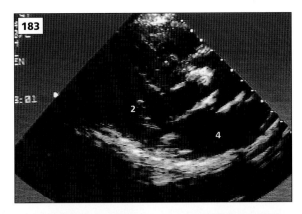

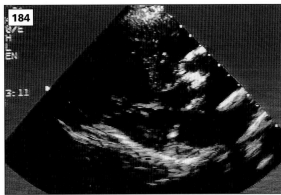

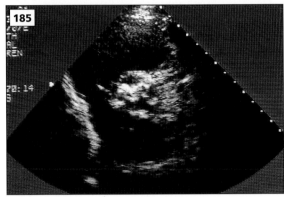

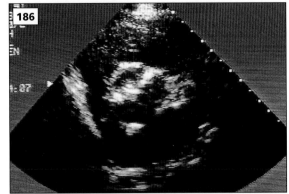

183–186. A very heavily calcified and immobile aortic valve in a slightly enlarged and calcified aortic root. In these two frames of the cardiac cycle there is almost no perceptible valvular movement. The left ventricular cavity is small and moderately hypertrophied, suggesting that there is significant left ventricular outflow tract obstruction. Short-axis parasternal views show this to be a degenerative three-cuspid valve with little motion in systole (**185,186**). In particular, there is calcification on the cuspal edges of the non-coronary cusp. There is little movement seen in the systolic frame (**186**). Apical continuous-wave Doppler interrogation shows there to be an increased velocity with a peak of >5 m/s, indicating severe stenosis (see **191**). The myocardium is at least 2 cm in thickness. The presence of severe left ventricular hypertrophy with a normal-sized cavity is suggestive of significant aortic stenosis. 2, LV; 4, LA.

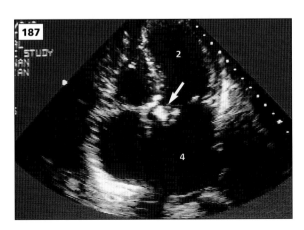

187. The aortic valve, particularly in the elderly, may become extremely heavily calcified with no obvious movement. The gradients across these valves may become large, though subsequent reduction in the gradient may occur with deterioration in left ventricular contraction. In this example, the valve is a mass of calcification with no perceivable movement of cusps (arrow). These are often best perceived in the apical five-chamber view. 2, LV; 4, LA.

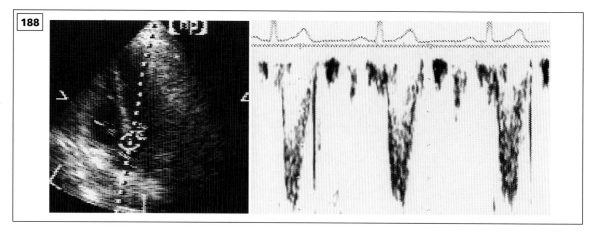

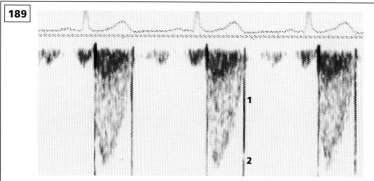

188–191. To obtain the maximum aortic gradient it is often necessary to interrogate the aortic valve from a number of planes to make certain the maximum velocity is recorded. Normal pulsed-wave Doppler recording from the apex showing a velocity of <1 m/s across a normal aortic valve (**188**). Mild aortic stenosis (**189**) showing the opening and closing movement of the valve with a velocity of approximately 2 m/s. As the aortic stenosis becomes more severe the blood flow velocity increases. In this case (**190**) it is approximately 3.5 m/s, suggesting a valve gradient of between 40 and 50 mmHg. In addition, there is mild aortic regurgitation. In this case of severe aortic stenosis (**191**) peak velocities of >5 m/s (transvalvular gradient >125 mmHg) are obtained from apical continuous-wave Doppler interrogation.

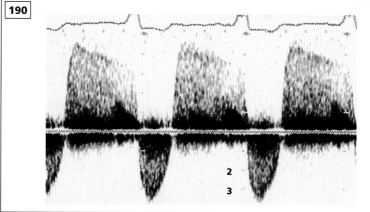

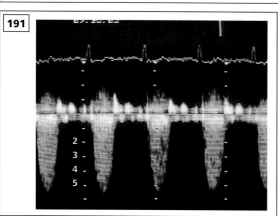

Transvalvular gradients obtained at cardiac catheterization and from Doppler are often compared. It is important to remember that these techniques measure different parameters. Doppler measures the true peak instantaneous pressure difference between the left ventricle and aorta. At catheterization, the peak-to-peak gradient is usually measured, i.e. not a true physiological measurement. The peak instantaneous pressure gradient is greater than the peak-to-peak gradient by about 20 mmHg, but the difference can be as much as 50 mmHg. The natural history of aortic valve disease has been derived from catheter studies.

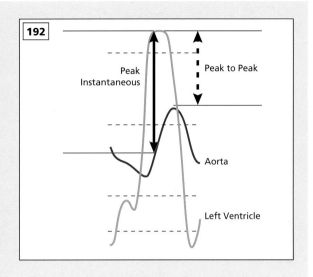

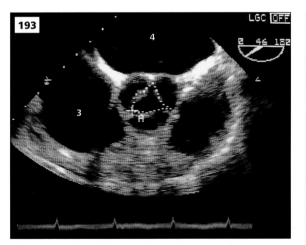

193. Direct planimetry of the aortic orifice area may be performed at transesophageal echocardiography. Calcification of the aortic leaflets and posterior aortic root may distort the orifice and affect the accuracy of this method. The valve area of this patient measured 1.8 cm² (see dotted line outlining orifice). 3, RA; 4, LA.

- In elderly patients, if the aortic valve appears to open it is unlikely to be severely stenosed.

- There is an approximate relationship between the degree of left ventricular hypertrophy (LVH) and the severity of aortic stenosis. In particular, it is unlikely that significant aortic obstruction will exist in the absence of LVH.

- Assessment of the severity of aortic obstruction in the presence of significantly impaired left ventricular function may be very difficult. While calculation of the transvalvular gradient usually suffices for clinical decision making, in this situation calculation of the valve area by the continuity equation is more helpful. The normal aortic valve area is 2.5–4.5 cm²: a valve area of 0.8 cm² represents severe stenosis, >0.8–1.0 cm² moderate stenosis, and >1.1 cm² only mild narrowing.

Aortic Regurgitation

There are various Doppler and imaging methods for assessing the severity of aortic regurgitation. The simplest relates to left ventricular function and dilatation as the larger the left ventricle, the more severe the aortic regurgitation, unless there is impairment of left ventricular contraction. Color-flow Doppler is very sensitive at detecting the presence of aortic regurgitation but, at present, the information obtained is related to velocity not volume, therefore does not assess severity. The pulsed-wave Doppler can be used to map the length (and how far it extends backwards into the left ventricle) of the regurgitant jet and continuous-wave Doppler traces of the regurgitant jet bear some relationship to the severity of regurgitation. In principle, the steeper the diastolic slope of the continuous-wave trace, the more severe the aortic regurgitation (as the left ventricular–aortic gradient at end-diastole is least).

Causes of aortic regurgitation are listed in *Table 8*; assessment by Doppler echocardiography of the severity of aortic regurgitation is shown in *Table 9*.

- *Clinical findings may provide a clue to the etiology of aortic regurgitation. Coexistent mitral valve disease suggests a rheumatic etiology, a Marfanoid habitus may indicate aortic ectasia, and an ejection click a bicuspid aortic valve.*

- *The chest radiograph may also be helpful, as a widened mediastinum suggests aortic root dilatation or dissection.*

Table 8. Causes of aortic regurgitation	
Valvular	**Acquired** Calcific degeneration Rheumatic fever Bacterial endocarditis **Congenital** Bicuspid valve Aortic valve prolapse Associated with membranous VSD

Aortic root	**Dilatation**
	Medial necrosis
	  Idiopathic
	  Hypertension
	  Old age
	Collagen abnormalities
	  Marfan's syndrome
	  Ehlers–Danlos syndrome
	  Osteogenesis imperfecta
	Inflammatory disorders
	  Rheumatoid arthritis
	  Systemic lupus erythematosus
	  Reiter's syndrome
	  Giant cell arteritis
	  Syphilis
	  Ankylosing spondylitis
	
	Aneurysm
	
	Dissection
	
	Trauma

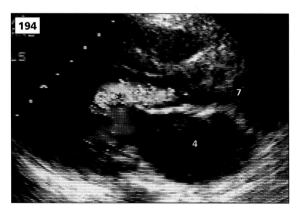

194. Parasternal long-axis echocardiogram showing mild aortic regurgitation. There is a moderately wide but short jet of aortic regurgitation (*) from a normal-looking valve without root dilatation. The left ventricle is of normal size and contraction. Many normal individuals, particularly those aged over 75, show some degree of aortic regurgitation which is not hemodynamically significant. 4, LA; 7, AO.

Table 9. Assessment of severity of aortic regurgitation by Doppler	
Jet measurements	Jet length and area – imperfect relationship to severity • *wall adherent jets underestimated (Coanda effect)* • *mixing with mitral inflow (coflow) can obscure area* Jet width in LVOT – easier to define than jet length • *jet width should be related to outflow tract diameter* • *ratio >60% implies severe aortic regurgitation*
Regurgitant orifice size	Cross-sectional area of jet at its origin – still experimental
Spectral Doppler	**Diastolic pressure decay rates** • In severe aortic regurgitation the slope of the continuous wave Doppler signal is steep reflecting the rapid equalization of left ventricular and aortic pressures. The pressure half-time is short (<400 ms) **Quantitative measurements** • Regurgitant volume = (LVOT area × LVOT VTI) – (Pulm area × Pulm VTI) • Regurgitant fraction = Regurgitant volume ÷ (LVOT area × LVOT VTI) ×100 • Regurgitant orifice area = Regurgitant volume ÷ Regurgitant VTI **Retrograde diastolic flow in descending aorta** • Continuous reversed flow through diastole implies significant aortic regurgitation LVOT = left ventricular outflow tract Pulm = pulmonary VTI = velocity time integral

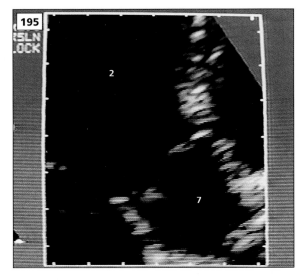

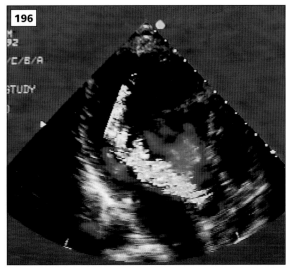

195, 196. Prolapse of one leaflet of a bicuspid valve is one cause of aortic regurgitation which occurs in childhood and adolescence. Most bicuspid aortic valves become stenotic, but some become predominantly regurgitant. In this example, there is a bicuspid aortic valve which opens widely and is not stenotic. Color flow (**196**) shows there is a jet of regurgitation arising from the cusp of the more posterior of the leaflets. The apical two-chamber view shows that the long jet arises centrally and tracks back into the left ventricle towards the apex. In this example, the left ventricle is not dilated or hyperdynamic, suggesting that the degree of regurgitation is no more than moderate. This would correspond to an aortographic severity of 2–3. 2, LV; 7, AO.

- *Serial assessment of ventricular size is a very helpful parameter in aortic regurgitation. Progressive cavity enlargement is probably evidence for early valve replacement.*

- *When assessing a patient with aortic regurgitation, it is vital to assess the ascending region and arch of the aorta, as in many aortic diseases it is the primary cause of regurgitation or has dilated as a secondary event.*

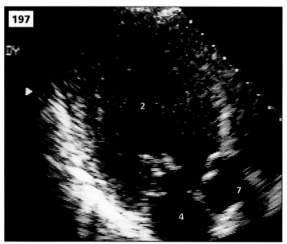

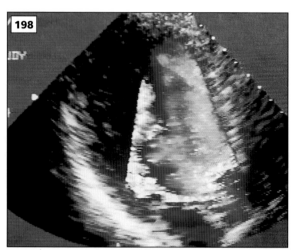

197, 198. With increasing severity of aortic regurgitation, the valve itself may still look normal. In this case, there is a bicuspid valve without root dilatation (**197**). The jet of aortic regurgitation is narrow but reaches more than

half-way to the apex of the left ventricle. The angle of the jet is across the anterior leaflet of the mitral valve and this may produce abnormal motion of this structure. 2, LV; 4, LA; 7, AO.

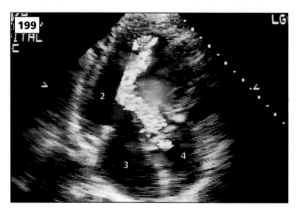

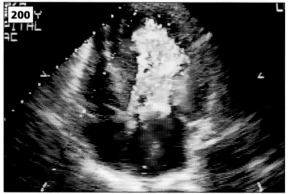

199, 200. Imaging of the color jet of aortic regurgitation may look different in different planes. Comparing a two- and four-chamber view of the same patient, the jet is a

good deal wider and longer in the latter, and this may suggest that regurgitation is more severe. 2, LV; 3, RA; 4, LA.

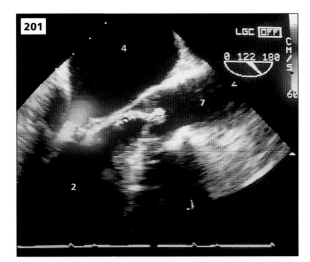

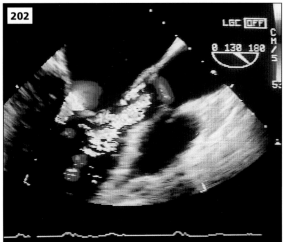

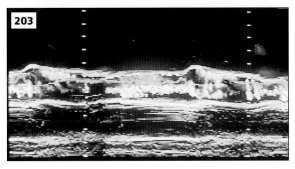

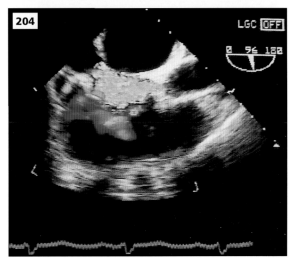

201–204. The transesophageal echocardiogram (120° plane) may demonstrate the presence of aortic regurgitation and establish its cause. In these examples there are increasing degrees of severity of aortic regurgitation as determined by color maps. The width of the aortic regurgitant jet in the left ventricular outflow tract is considered to be related to severity of regurgitation. Figure (**201**) shows a tiny narrow jet of insignificant aortic regurgitation. Moderate aortic regurgitation is seen as a wider jet (**202**) and the corresponding color M-mode echocardiography confirms that the jet is holodiastolic but does not fill the outflow tract (**203**). In severe aortic regurgitation the entire outflow tract is filled by a color regurgitant jet (**204**). 2, LV; 4, LA; 7, AO.

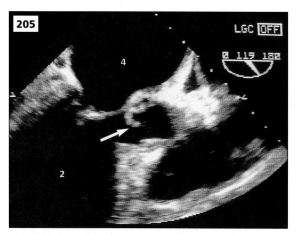

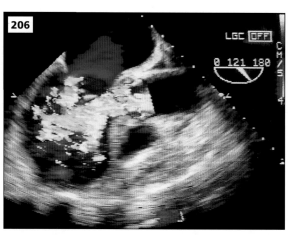

205, 206. In patients without root dilatation the regurgitation is not usually central, but through a cusp rupture. In this transesophageal example in the 120° plane the cusp prolapse is seen (arrow) (**205**) and the color jet of severe regurgitation arises centrally in a region of perforation of the cusp due to infective endocarditis (**206**). 2, LV; 4, LA.

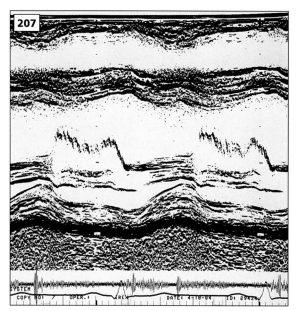

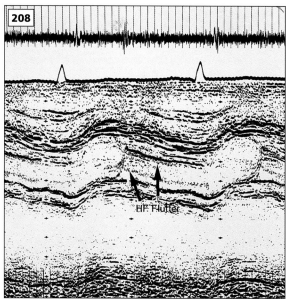

207. The M-mode echocardiogram is often unhelpful in the assessment of the cause of aortic regurgitation. It may, of course, be very useful to determine the presence of mitral valve flutter, which is not easily seen by cross-sectional echocardiography because of the lower frame rate. The presence of mitral valve flutter is not pathognomonic of the presence of aortic regurgitation, although it is a useful subsidiary finding. The size of the left ventricle is best measured by M-mode echocardiography and, as discussed above, bears a strong relationship to the severity of regurgitation and the need for surgery.

208. Occasionally, when there is a perforated aortic leaflet, flutter may be seen on the aortic valve. Because of the low frame rate of cross-sectional systems, one can only visualize the systolic flutter of aortic leaflets by conventional M-mode echocardiography.

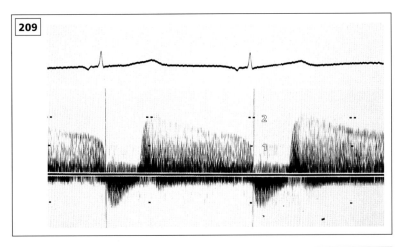

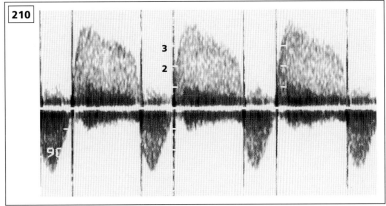

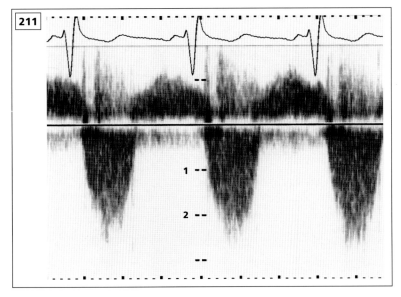

209–211. Doppler ultrasound may be used for the semi-quantitative assessment of aortic regurgitation. A variety of equations is available but probably those of any clinical importance are related to the diastolic slope of the continuous-wave trace. *Table 9* details the various methods that have been put forward as of use. The apical trace shown is of trivial aortic regurgitation (**209**). There is no increase in forward velocities (below the line) and the slope in diastole is shallow, representing a persistent aortic–left ventricular gradient, even at the end of diastole. In severe aortic regurgitation (**210**), as shown, the slope is much more significant and when severe or acute, there may be no aortic–left ventricular gradient. Of course, as the left ventricular end-diastolic pressure rises, this may become the limiting factor in aortic pressure and therefore, there will be no Doppler flow in end-diastole. In addition, reversal of the blood flow velocities in the descending aorta is a measure of severity (**211**). Occasionally, there may be considerable discrepancies between the measurement of aortic gradients by the Bernoulli equation. This may occur when there is severe aortic regurgitation and mild aortic stenosis. The increased blood volume crossing the abnormal aortic valve may increase the blood velocity, leading to spurious high gradients.

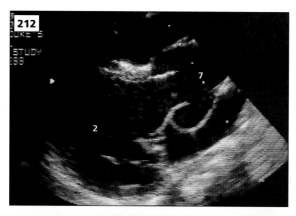

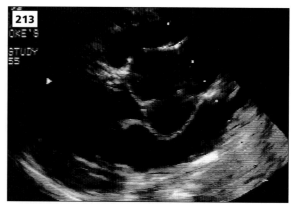

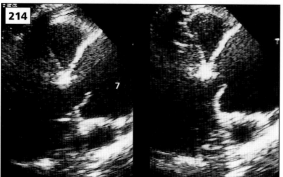

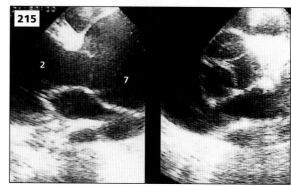

212–215. Aortic root disease is the most common form of aortic regurgitation in the west. This is usually associated with a forme fruste of Marfan's syndrome. Other causes of aortic root dilatation are extensive and are often associated with connective tissue disorders. Systolic (**212**) and diastolic (**213**) frames are shown in a child with Marfan's syndrome. The aortic root size is related to height and in this 4-year-old, there is obvious dilatation of the Sinuses of Valsalva, though the valve itself appears to function relatively normally. With increasing severity of aortic dilatation, there is eventual failure of coaptation and central regurgitation. The root dilatation may be of a fusiform or saccular type. Of the former type (**214**), there is a huge aortic root with a valve failing to coapt, which is more typical of Marfan's syndrome. In contrast, the saccular type (**215**) shows on cross-sectional views that though the valve is stretched across this dilated annulus, the root is not particularly large as the dilatation arises above this area. 2, LV; 7, AO.

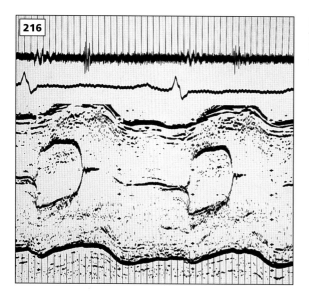

216. The M-mode echocardiogram is useful for measuring the size of the aortic root. In this example, the aortic root is 6 cm and the aortic valve is shown opening normally within this large structure.

7 AORTIC VALVE REPLACEMENT

Aortic valve replacement may be undertaken for stenosis and/or regurgitation and, less commonly, for infection and aortic dissection. Left ventricular structure and function postoperatively depends on the preoperative lesion. Early postoperative ventricular septal motion is paradoxical and it may be difficult to assess left ventricular contraction. In severe pre-operative aortic regurgitation and stenosis there may be quite marked postoperative left ventricular hypertrophy which takes a considerable period – perhaps up to one year – to regress fully. Despite poor left ventricular contraction preoperatively, even in the presence of pulmonary edema, patients with aortic stenosis have at least a moderate degree of recovery of function. In contrast, patients with impaired left ventricular contraction and dilatation due to aortic regurgitation often show no significant recovery.

The variety of aortic valve replacements in current use – both biological and mechanical – is listed in *Table 10*. Echocardiographic features of biological aortic valve replacements are shown in *Table 11*.

Table 10. Aortic valve replacements
Biological
Autograft (pulmonary to aortic switch)
Homograft (unstented) cadaveric aortic and pulmonary valves
Xenograft porcine aortic valve: • Carpentier–Edwards • Hancock bovine pericardium: Ionescu–Shiley
Mechanical
Ball and cage: Starr–Edwards
Single tilting disc: • Björk–Shiley • Hall–Medtronics • Lillehei–Kaster • Omniscience
Bileaflet: • St Jude Medical • Carbomedics • Duromedics

Table 11. Doppler parameters in normal aortic bioprostheses			
	Peak velocity (m/s)	**Peak gradient** (mmHg)	**Mean gradient** (mmHg)
Carpentier–Edwards (porcine valve)	2.5 ± 0.5	23.2 ± 8.7	14.4 ± 5.7
Hancock (porcine valve)	2.4 ± 0.4	23.0 ± 6.7	11.0 ± 2.3
Ionescu–Shiley (pericardial valve)	2.5 ± 1.7	24.7 ± 7.7	14.0 ± 4.3

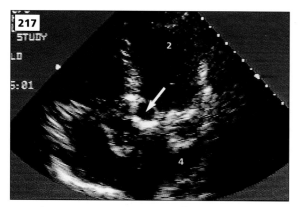

217. The normal aortic xenograft has thin mobile cusps but usually degenerates by becoming calcified and initially stenotic. In a similar fashion to the mitral prosthesis, the valve eventually becomes rigid and loses its structural integrity and often becomes acutely and severely regurgitant. In an apical five-chamber view, the valve is seen as a calcified mass with no perceptible movement (arrow). There is an increase in blood flow velocity with a peak velocity of approximately 4 m/s across this valve. 2, LV; 4, LA.

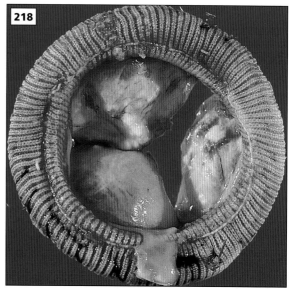

218. A pathologic specimen in this type of degeneration shows calcified masses on the ventricular aspect of the xenograft.

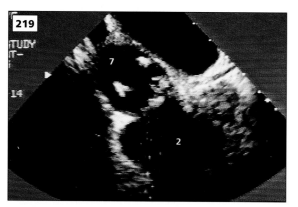

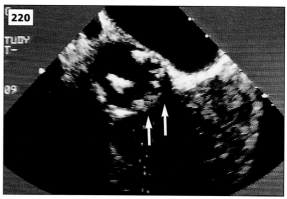

219, 220. Two frames of a transesophageal echocardiogram with a prolapsing and severely regurgitant aortic xenograft. The valve is seen to be prolapsing into the left ventricular outflow tract (arrows). This valve is thickened and there is no evidence of vegetation suggesting endocarditis. 2, LV; 7, AO.

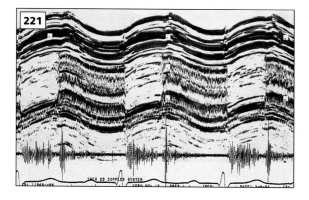

221. The M-mode echocardiogram may show fluttering of a perforated xenograft cusp in diastole.

Imaging echocardiography is often unhelpful in examining mechanical prostheses. *Table 12* shows the echocardiographic features of mechanical aortic valve replacements. Doppler examination may demonstrate stenosis or regurgitation. Often, the transesophageal echocardiogram will reveal any significant abnormality.

With all prosthetic valve replacements, imaging of the leaflets is usually inadequate for accurate assessment. However, valve leaflet motion can usually be detected. More useful is the color Doppler detection of a paraprosthetic leak or abnormal valve motion. As the subaortic velocity is similar to the transaortic velocity, the simplified Bernoulli equation is less accurate than in native aortic stenosis and can lead to overdiagnosis of obstruction. The full modified Bernoulli equation should be employed to diagnose the transaortic gradient across prosthetic valves.

Table 12.
Doppler parameters in normal mechanical aortic prostheses

	Peak velocity (m/s)	**Peak gradient** (mmHg)	**Mean gradient** (mmHg)
Starr–Edwards	3.2 ± 0.6	38.6 ± 11.7	23.0 ± 8.0
St Jude Medical	2.4 ± 0.3	25.5 ± 5.1	12.5 ± 6.4
Björk–Shiley	2.5 ± 0.6	23.8 ± 8.8	14.3 ± 5.3

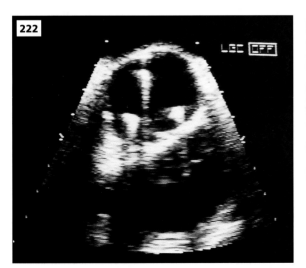

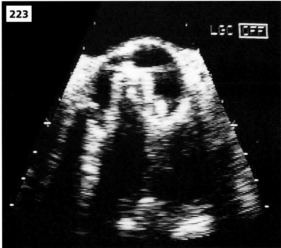

222, 223. Transesophageal transverse plane image of a normally functioning Starr–Edwards prosthesis. Three dense struts are seen in systole (**222**) and the ball is seen in diastole (**223**). Such valves often have a Doppler gradient across them. In a small valve, e.g. one less than 21 mm, there may be a Doppler flow velocities of 3–4 m/s.

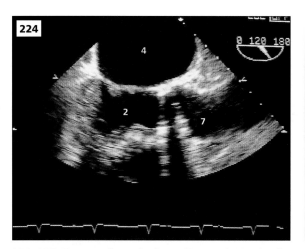

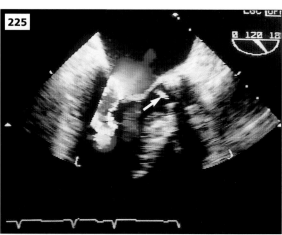

224, 225. Transesophageal echocardiogram (120° plane) in a normally functioning bileaflet St Jude tilting disc valve which shows the two discs opening normally in systole (**224**). Shadowing from the discs obscures the left ventricular outflow tract to an extent but the color-flow image (**225**) demonstrates a whiff of aortic regurgitation which is normal for this valve (arrow). This patient also had mitral stenosis. 2, LV; 4, LA; 7, AO.

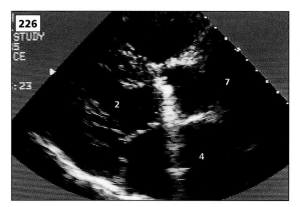

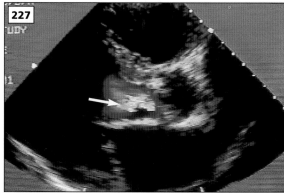

226, 227. Parasternal long-axis view of a Bjork–Shiley aortic valve replacement in which moderate paraprosthetic regurgitation (**227**) has occurred. The left ventricle is hypertrophied and hyperdynamic. Little detail is obtained by imaging the valve directly because of the masking due to reverberation. A discrete color-flow jet of aortic regurgitation (arrow) is seen arising posteriorly due to partial dehiscence of the sewing ring. 2, LV; 4, LA; 7, AO.

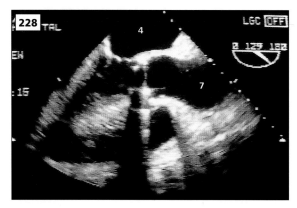

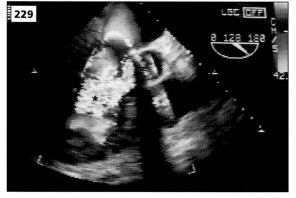

228, 229. Transesophageal echocardiography (120° plane) in a patient with severe paraprosthetic aortic regurgitation following a bileaflet Carbomedics aortic valve replacement. No defect is visualized but the color-flow view (**229**) shows a severe paraprosthetic aortic regurgitant jet (*). 4, LA; 7, AO.

8 SUB- and SUPRA-AORTIC STENOSIS

Subaortic Stenosis

Discrete subaortic stenosis may occur as an isolated lesion or more commonly in the presence of other congenital heart disease, particularly ventricular septal and atrioventricular septal defect and aortic stenosis. While it may be difficult to differentiate the clinical features of aortic stenosis, hypertrophic cardiomyopathy and subaortic stenosis, this diagnosis is usually readily apparent by echo-cardiography. Typical features are of a membrane or more substantial structure in the left ventricular outflow tract. This may be associated with abnormality of the anterior leaflet of the mitral valve. The obstruction in this area leads to increased blood flow velocity on Doppler and turbulent blood flow by color imaging. The aortic valve may open in an unusual pattern with mid-systolic closure and flutter. The degree of obstruction may be assessed in a similar way to valvular aortic stenosis by continuous-wave Doppler and assessment of left ventricular hypertrophy. This obstruction may be dynamic and increase with Valsalva maneuvers and extrasystoles (see Hypertrophic cardiomyopathy, p. 121).

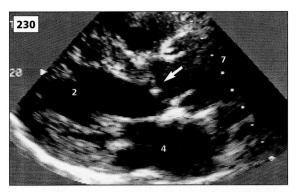

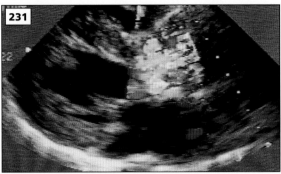

230, 231. Severe subaortic stenosis due to a membranous structure (arrow) lying below a normal-looking aortic valve. There was a turbulent area of blood flow and an increase in blood flow velocity to 5 m/s. There is severe left ventricular hypertrophy. 2, LV; 4, LA; 7, AO.

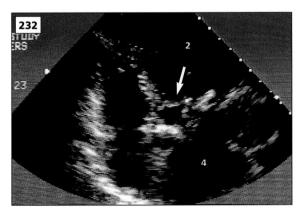

232. The subaortic obstruction (arrow) is often best seen in apical five-chamber views as in this example where there is thickening of the aortic valve as well. To obtain a Doppler outflow tract velocity, the five-chamber view is most appropriate. 2, LV; 4, LA.

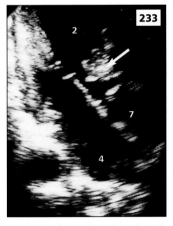

233. Apical two-chamber view showing subaortic obstruction of the tunnel variety. This is a mixture of fibrous tissue and muscle (arrow) and often leads to very severe left ventricular hypertrophy. It is occasionally difficult to differentiate this form of subaortic stenosis from localized septal hypertrophy with outflow tract obstruction in hypertrophic cardiomyopathy. 2, LV; 4, LA; 7, AO.

In patients with a systolic murmur and left ventricular hypertrophy it is important to actively exclude a subaortic obstruction. This may only be seen in one view and often the apical long-axis view (right anterior oblique equivalent) is the most helpful. Occasionally in patients with a diagnosis of hypertrophic cardiomyopathy, the left ventricular outflow tract in not narrowed between the septum and anterior mitral leaflet, but a discrete membrane may be seen with transesophageal echocardiography.

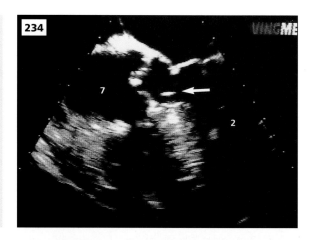

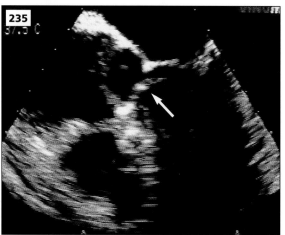

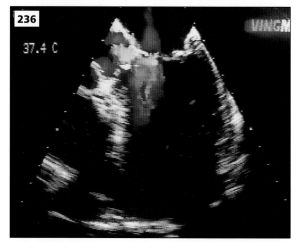

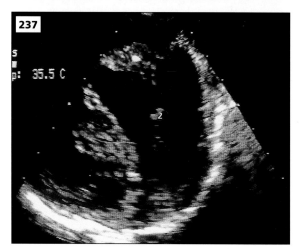

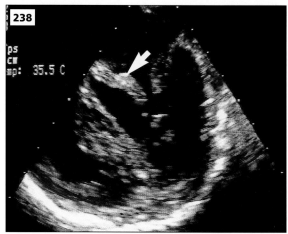

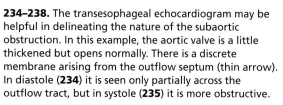

234–238. The transesophageal echocardiogram may be helpful in delineating the nature of the subaortic obstruction. In this example, the aortic valve is a little thickened but opens normally. There is a discrete membrane arising from the outflow septum (thin arrow). In diastole (**234**) it is seen only partially across the outflow tract, but in systole (**235**) it is more obstructive.

Color-flow imaging in systole (**236**) shows this to be the site of obstruction. There is severe left ventricular hypertrophy with a small left ventricular cavity (**237**) and the mitral valve is myxomatous (**238**) (fat arrow) which is a common accompaniment of subaortic stenosis. 2, LV; 7, AO.

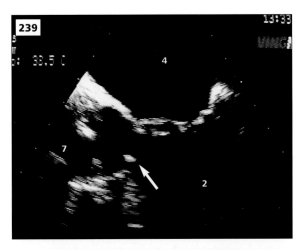

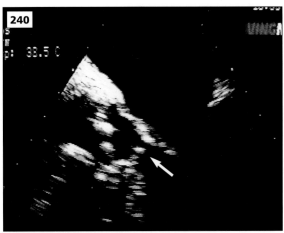

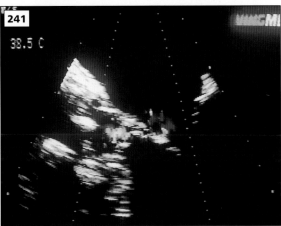

239–241. The subaortic stenosis may coexist with aortic valve disease and be difficult to identify. This has important implications in the postoperative period if missed, as the inotropes used in the post-surgical period may exacerbate the outflow tract gradient. The subaortic membrane (arrow) needs to be differentiated from the muscle bulge which is seen in the outflow tract ventricular septum in left ventricular hypertrophy, particularly where there is increased angulation between the septum and aortic root. This is described under Normal Variants (pp. 16–24). In this example, there is a membrane (arrow) lying below the aortic valve attached to the ventricular septum which is only partially obstructed (**239**). The aortic valve is thickened and obstructive (**240**). In diastole, the membrane lies in contact with the anterior leaflet of the mitral valve (arrow). An area of turbulent blood flow is seen in this area in systole (**241**). 2, LV; 4, LA; 7, AO.

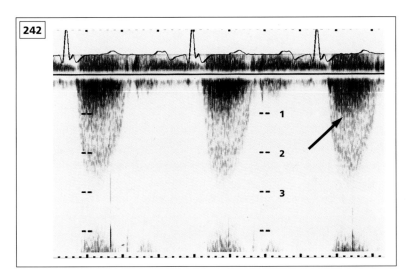

242. Continuous-wave Doppler examination from the apex in moderate severity subaortic stenosis. The peak velocity approaches 3 m/s. While there is a clear envelope, there is also an underlying trace suggesting a normal (>1 m/s) flow across the aortic valve (arrow).

Supra-Aortic Stenosis

This is an unusual form of left ventricular outflow tract obstruction and is usually seen in infants with other congenital diseases including William's syndrome. It is often difficult to localize the proximal ascending aorta by ultrasound but it is probably best achieved in angulated parasternal long-axis views.

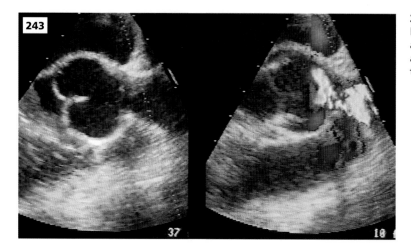

243. Supravalvar aortic stenosis. The left hand image shows a normal aortic valve with a discrete waist above the sinuses of Valsalva with turbulent flow on color map (right).

- Although uncommon, supravalvular aortic stenosis occurs with sufficient frequency to merit consideration in the diagnosis of left ventricular outflow obstruction.

- The most frequent type is the hourglass deformity characterized by extreme thickening of the media of the ascending aorta. Less common are the membranous type of a fibrous diaphragm with a single perforation and the hypoplastic type comprising uniform hypoplasia of the entire ascending aorta.

9 TRICUSPID VALVE DISEASE

The most common tricuspid lesion is simple regurgitation. With modern Doppler and color-flow imaging systems, tricuspid regurgitation may be demonstrated in normal individuals. With any form of raised pulmonary artery pressure, tricuspid regurgitation is frequently seen. The ability to measure right ventricular systolic pressure from the tricuspid regurgitant jet velocity has been a major advance. Frequently, tricuspid regurgitation is associated with a normal valvular anatomy. The causes of tricuspid valve disease are listed in *Table 13*.

Echocardiography is not particularly effective at assessing the severity of tricuspid regurgitation. A semi-quantitative approach can be achieved by analyzing the length and width of regurgitant jets and by mapping the regurgitant jet back from the valve into the great veins.

Pulmonary artery systolic pressure may be reliably estimated using the peak systolic velocity of the tricuspid regurgitant jet. The peak jet velocity allows calculation of the right atrial to right ventricular systolic pressure gradient from the Bernoulli formula ($4V^2$). Addition of this gradient to the right atrial pressure (measured directly by central venous line or estimated as 5–10 mmHg) will give the peak systolic right ventricular pressure. In the absence of pulmonary stenosis this will equal the pulmonary artery systolic pressure.

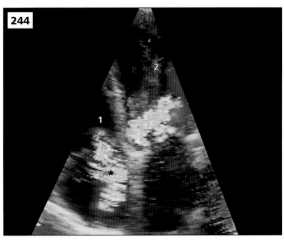

244. Mild tricuspid regurgitation in a patient with left-sided valvar disease, including aortic and mitral regurgitation. The tricuspid valve appears structurally normal, though there is a central jet of regurgitation (*) of less than 3 m/s. This would suggest that the right ventricular pressure is not significantly elevated. As right ventricular pressure becomes higher, tricuspid annular dilatation may be seen. 1, RV; 2, LV.

Table 13. Causes of tricuspid valve disease
Functional tricuspid regurgitation
Rheumatic
Myxomatous degeneration
Infective endocarditis
Congenital e.g. Ebstein's anomaly
Carcinoid
Rare SLE Endomyocardial fibrosis

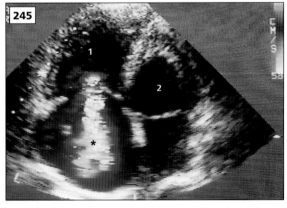

245. In severe pulmonary hypertension the annulus is dilated and there is a long but narrow central jet of tricuspid regurgitation (*) with a velocity across this of 4 m/s (suggesting a right ventricular systolic pressure of 64 mmHg). An area of flow convergence is seen on the ventricular aspect of the tricuspid valve. 1, RV; 2, LV.

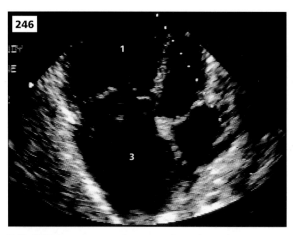

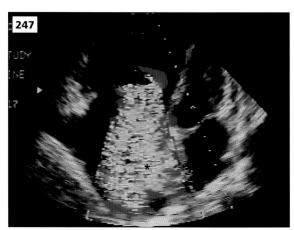

246, 247. In pulmonary hypertension where the pulmonary artery pressure may exceed the systemic pressure, the right ventricle becomes enlarged and hypertrophied and the tricuspid annulus dilated (**246**).

In comparison with the above figure (**245**), in this example there is a broad jet of tricuspid regurgitation filling the right atrium (*). 1, RV; 3, RA.

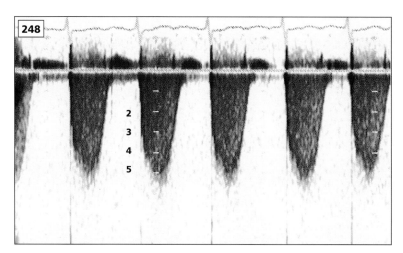

248. Continuous-wave Doppler examination of the tricuspid regurgitation jet. The peak velocity exceeds 5 m/s, suggesting systemic right ventricular pressures.

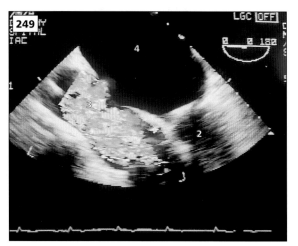

249. Transesophageal echocardiography transverse plane four-chamber view showing gross tricuspid regurgitation in a patient with mitral stenosis. 2, LV; 3, RA; 4, LA.

Ebstein's anomaly

In Ebstein's anomaly there is atrialization of the right ventricle with downward displacement of one or more leaflets of the tricuspid valve into the ventricle leading to an enlargement of the right atrium and tricuspid regurgitation.

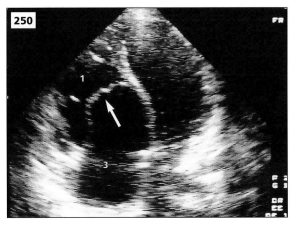

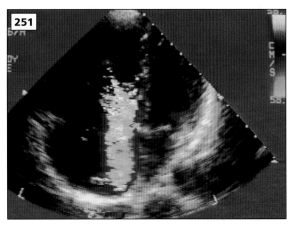

250, 251. These show the tricuspid valve as being attached down the ventricular septum from the normal annulus. In another example the tricuspid regurgitant jet is seen to arise further into the ventricular cavity than normal (**251**). The tricuspid valve in Ebstein's anomaly has an abnormal motion and there often appears to be a great deal of redundant tissue. 1, RV; 3, RA.

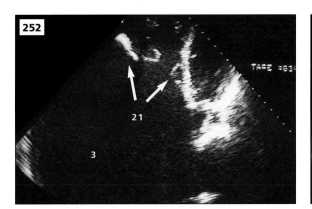

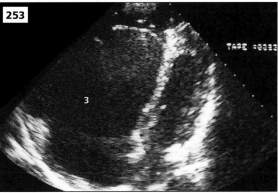

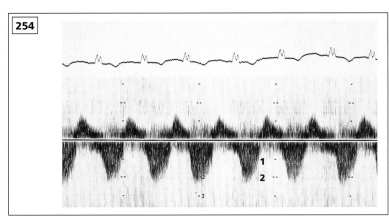

252–254. In Ebstein's anomaly the right atrium may become grossly enlarged, with the rest of the heart appearing as an appendage from it! In this example, it is difficult to appreciate any particular cardiac anatomy because of the distension of the right atrium. The Doppler traces in Ebstein's anomaly (**254**) show a jet of tricuspid regurgitation which is of low velocity because it is unusual to have accompanying pulmonary hypertension. 3, RA; 21, TV.

Tricuspid stenosis

Tricuspid stenosis is an uncommon accompaniment of rheumatic mitral valve disease. Very occasionally, tricuspid valve stenosis may occur due to other forms of obstruction such as tumor or thrombus.

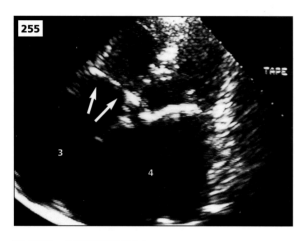

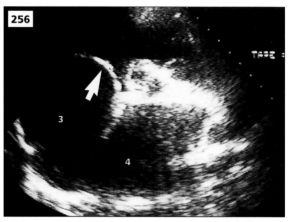

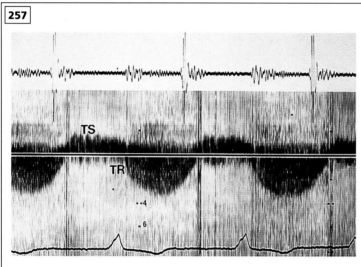

255–257. The tricuspid valve can often be difficult to image when stenotic. In the first example, in an apical four-chamber view, a heavily calcified rheumatic mitral valve is seen with an enlarged left atrium (**255**). In addition, the tricuspid valve is a rigid domed structure (thin arrows). In short-axis parasternal views in a different patient (**256**), the domed nature of this valve can be seen (fat arrow). Since there are difficulties in diagnosing tricuspid stenosis with hemodynamic traces, continuous-wave Doppler interpretation may be the method of choice for documenting obstruction to this valve. In this example, there is an increase in blood flow velocity with a slow diastolic decline. In addition, there is tricuspid regurgitation (**257**). 3, RA; 4, LA.

- Measurement of transvalvular gradient by Doppler is probably the best method by which to assess the severity of tricuspid stenosis. Mean gradients correlate well with invasive haemodynamic measurements.

- The pressure half-time method is unsuitable as the appropriate constant for the tricuspid valve has not been determined.

Carcinoid syndrome

Carcinoid syndrome is caused by the release of 5-hydroxytryptamine from a metastasizing carcinoid tumor. The primary tumor usually is found in the gastrointestinal tract and carcinoid tumors of the ileum are most likely to metastasize. Clinical manifestations of this syndrome are related to the circulation of serotonin and other humoral substances; they include flushing, diarrhea and wheezing.

Carcinoid tumors that metastasize to the liver result in carcinoid heart disease, as the liver fails to inactivate the tumor products, which then reach the heart in large quantities. In over 50% of patients fibrotic damage occurs to the tricuspid and pulmonary valves and results in tricuspid regurgitation and pulmonary stenosis. The right atrium and right ventricle frequently are dilated. Left heart involvement is rare (except with bronchial carcinoid tumors), presumably because the tumor products are inactivated by the lungs. If suspected, carcinoid syndrome usually can be confirmed by measurement of the serotonin metabolite 5-hydroxyindoleacetic acid in a 24 hour urinary collection.

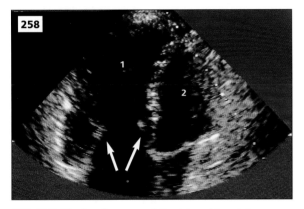 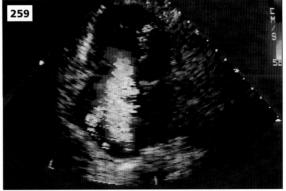

258, 259. The involvement of the tricuspid and, to a lesser extent, pulmonary valves by carcinoid syndrome is readily demonstrated by ultrasound. The tricuspid valve has a characteristic appearance. It is thickened and immobile and appears to be stuck in a half-open, half-closed position (arrows) (**258**). There is significant tricuspid regurgitation which may become gross as the disease progresses (**259**). 1, RV; 2, LV.

> *In an adult patient with isolated tricuspid or pulmonary valve disease the diagnosis of carcinoid should always be considered.*

Tricuspid Valve Replacement

Prosthetic valves in the tricuspid position may be assessed by transthoracic echo techniques. When transthoracic scans are inadequate, transeso-phageal imaging may yield further information on the tricuspid prosthetic valve structure and function.

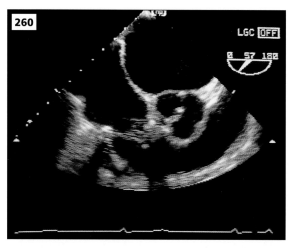

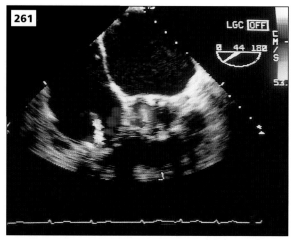

260, 261. Transesophageal echocardiography, transverse short-axis view, showing a tricuspid valve replacement with a small color-flow jet of mild tricuspid regurgitation (**261**).

- Tricuspid valve replacement is relatively rare.
- Doppler-derived tricuspid prosthetic valve gradients seem to correlate well with those measured invasively.

- Pressure half-times from normally functioning tricuspid valve prostheses are longer than those from mitral valve prostheses, but a pressure half-time of >200 ms and forward peak velocity of >1.6 m/s suggests significant stenosis.

10 INFECTIVE ENDOCARDITIS

Before the development of cardiac ultrasound, the demonstration of valvular vegetations was possible only at surgery and autopsy. Early in the development of the technique, it has been apparent that vegetations could be readily demonstrated on valves. Among patients with a definite diagnosis of endocarditis, approximately two-thirds will have vegetations demonstrated by transthoracic imaging. This percentage will rise to more than 90% when the imaging is carried out by the transesophageal route. The minimum size seen by transthoracic imaging is 3 mm and possibly 2 mm by transesophageal probes. The absence of vegetation does not exclude a diagnosis of endocarditis. Vegetations may be seen on the valves or attached to ruptured mitral valve chordae tendineae. Less frequently, valve perforation or abscess formation may be demonstrated. Serial echocardiography is important to demonstrate enlargement of vegetations, valve disruption and abscess formation. Occasionally, the diagnosis of vegetation may be confused by the presence of ruptured chordae tendineae, which vibrate and produce a mass-like echocardiographic image, and heavily calcified valves when the features of the valve anatomy are not clearly seen. Occasionally, a myxoma may arise from the valve itself, as may a number of other tumors (see Cardiac Masses, p. 87).

The aim of echocardiography in suspected infective endocarditis is to:

- *Diagnose vegetations.*
- *Assess complications, e.g. abscess formation, hemodynamic complications.*
- *Determine underlying diagnoses (one-third will have normal valves).*
- *Monitor therapy (weekly echocardiograms).*

- *The absence of vegetations does not exclude the diagnosis of endocarditis.*

- *The presence of vegetations in a patient with even atypical clinical findings makes the probability of endocarditis very high.*

- *Serial echocardiograms are vital in patients with endocarditis to detect the destructive complications as early as possible.*

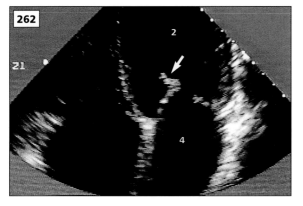

262. Mitral valve vegetations may vary in size and most commonly are attached to ruptured chordae. In this example, in an apical four-chamber view, a small mass is seen attached to a chorda on the anterior leaflet (arrow). To image the vegetation it may be necessary to view the area throughout the cardiac cycle and in several planes. 2, LV; 4, LA.

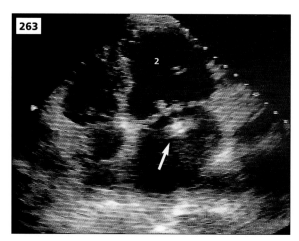

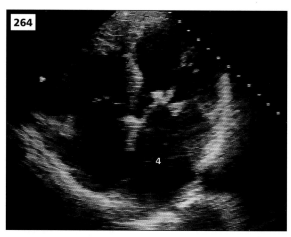

263, 264. As the vegetations become larger, they become more obvious. In this example, in systole (**263**), a large prolapsing mass is seen in the left atrium (arrow). This structure is vibrating rapidly in a regurgitant jet and tends to appear larger than its actual size. In this case, the left atrium is enlarged because of the severity of mitral regurgitation. In diastole (**264**), the mass prolapses through into the left ventricle. One can identify the areas of ruptured chordae as well as the redundant edge to the posterior leaflet. 2, LV; 4, LA.

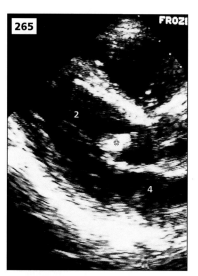

265. Vegetations may eventually become extremely large, as seen in this transthoracic parasternal view. A large vegetation (*) attached to a ruptured chorda tendinea is seen to prolapse into the left ventricular outflow tract during systole. 2, LV; 4, LA.

Vegetations shrink and become fibrotic and echodense with treatment, but they may not disappear altogether. Fresh vegetations tend to be less echodense and 'softer' in appearance.

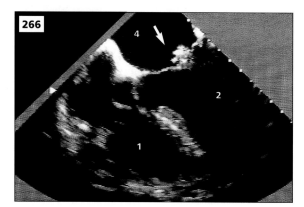

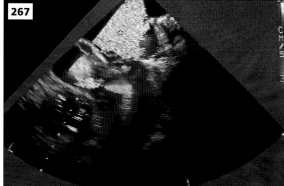

266, 267. Transesophageal echocardiography is particularly helpful in identifying small mitral valve vegetations (arrow). In this example, there is a 1 cm mass attached to the anterior leaflet of the mitral valve. Color-flow shows there to be severe mitral regurgitation with a broad jet of regurgitant flow filling the left atrium (*). This vegetation has disrupted mitral coaptation and led to acute regurgitation. 1, RV; 2, LV; 4, LA.

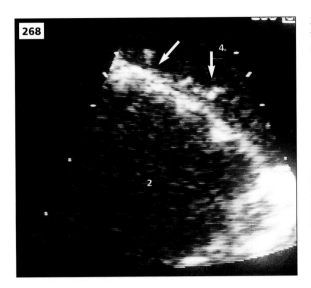

268. Transesophageal echocardiogram showing multiple vegetations on the atrial aspect of the mitral valve (arrows). 2, LV; 4, LA.

Because of the high resolution image obtained with transesophageal imaging, it is now believed that a negative scan in the presence of normal-looking native valves almost excludes endocarditis.

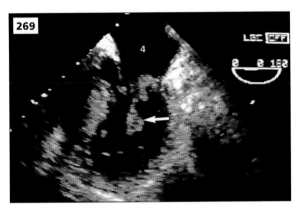

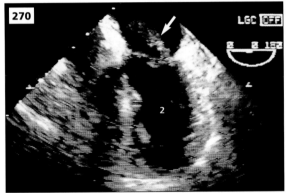

269, 270. Transesophageal echocardiogram showing a large friable mitral valve vegetation (arrows) prolapsing from left atrium to left ventricle. 2, LV; 4, LA.

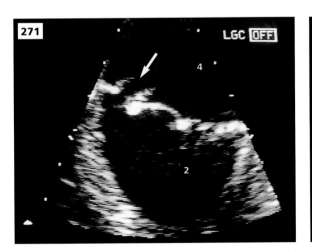

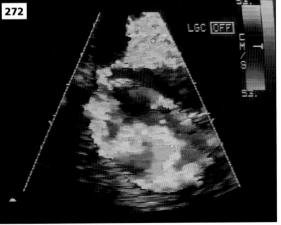

271, 272. Transesophageal echocardiogram showing a defect (arrow) with infected material in the anterior leaflet of the mitral valve with a color map showing severe mitral regurgitation through the perforation (*). 2, LV; 4, LA.

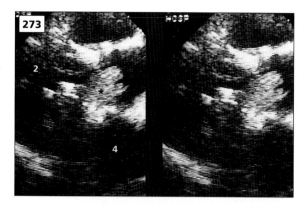

273. It may be possible to image vegetations on bioprostheses and these have a similar appearance, though tend to be more sessile than on native valves. It is unusual to see vegetations on mechanical valves by transthoracic echocardiography. However, on this example, there is a large mass (*) associated with a sewing ring of a Starr–Edwards mitral valve replacement. This is of fungal origin – hence its size – and tends to obstruct the left ventricular outflow tract. 2, LV; 4, LA.

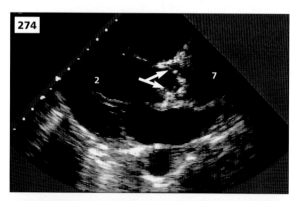

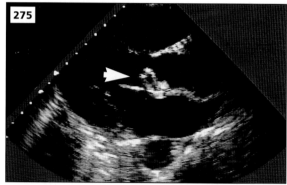

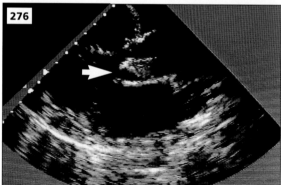

274–276. Endocarditis may occur on the basis of congenital aortic valve disease which is hemodynamically insignificant and less commonly seen on degenerative three-cuspid valves. In this example (parasternal long-axis view), there is a domed bicuspid valve (thin arrows) with a small vegetation sited on the posterior of these leaflets (fat arrows). During diastole, a structure associated with this leaflet is seen to prolapse progressively. This is a typical appearance of a vegetation which has disrupted a bicuspid valve. The aortic regurgitation associated with such vegetations is usually severe and rapidly progressive. 2, LV; 7, AO.

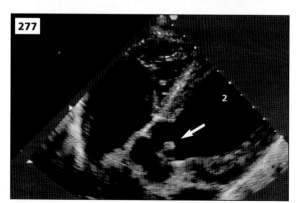

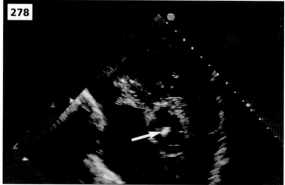

277, 278. To identify a valvular vegetation, it is imperative to image in all available planes, particularly if one is trying to exclude the diagnosis of endocarditis. In this example, the small aortic vegetation is only seen in subcostal views. This small defect of 2–3 mm is associated with a pedicle and can be seen (arrow) in both long- and short-axis views. 2, LV.

The differential diagnosis of a vegetation includes:

- A rolled-up ruptured chord.
- Redundant or torn cusp.
- Calcium.
- Thrombus.
- Valve tumors, including myxomas.
- Artifact, e.g. pacing electrodes or indwelling catheters.
- Lambl's excrescences.

A transesophageal study is required if:

- The transthoracic views are poor.
- The transthoracic study is normal but the clinical suspicion is high.
- There is suspected prosthetic valve endocarditis.
- There is suspected abscess.

Even if a transesophageal study is negative, in the presence of a highly suspicious clinical picture, it should repeated 1 week later, particularly in the presence of prosthetic valves.

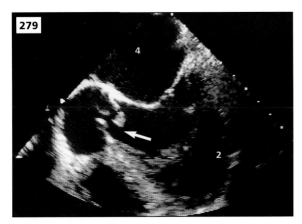

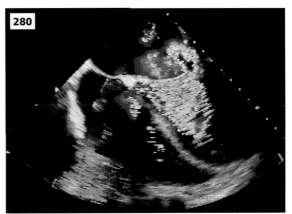

279, 280. Transesophageal imaging may give more anatomic detail concerning the valvular involvement in endocarditis. In this example, there is prolapse and perforation of the non-coronary leaflet (arrow) and color-flow shows a broad and long regurgitant jet. 2, LV; 4, LA.

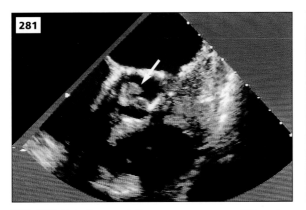

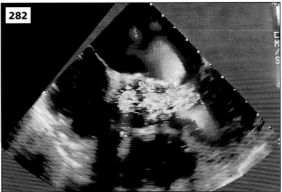

281, 282. Valvular vegetations may appear as different sizes, depending on the angle and route of imaging. For this reason, as described above, it is important to use every available window. In this example, aortic vegetations which appeared small by transthoracic views are, in fact, more than 1 cm in diameter on the transesophageal approach (arrow). This is associated with severe regurgitation. The size of the vegetation has important implications as surgery is much more likely to be needed when they are of a larger size.

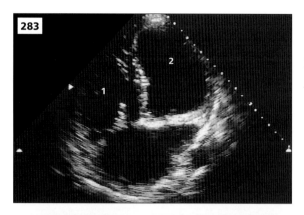

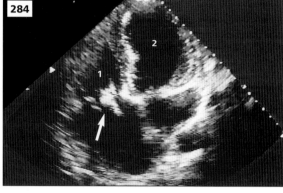

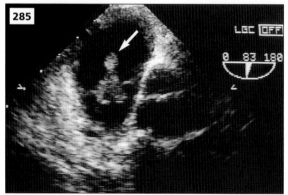

283–285. Much less commonly, other valves may be associated with endocarditis. In intravenous drug abusers, there is frequent association with infection of the tricuspid valve. Pacing wires and intravenous lines may very occasionally be the site of infection of the tricuspid valve. In this example (**283**) there is a small vegetation attached to ruptured chordae which appears much larger during a systolic cycle (arrow) (**284**) when it prolapses into the right atrium. A transesophageal echocardiogram (**285**) from a different patient shows a large tricuspid vegetation due to an indwelling venous line (arrow). 1, RV; 2, LV.

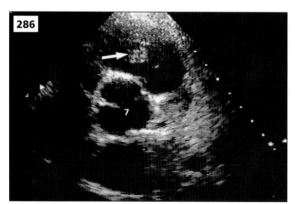

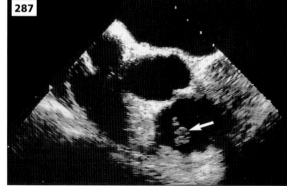

286, 287. Very rarely, patients who have had prolonged parenteral treatment with in-dwelling long lines may have infection of the right-sided valves. This is usually on the basis of a normal valve which has been traumatized by a catheter passing through it. In this example, a mass of approximately 1 cm is seen prolapsing into the right ventricular outflow tract from a thin pulmonary valve (**286**, arrow). Transesophageal imaging (**287**) shows this to be ejected into the pulmonary artery during systole (arrow). 7, AO.

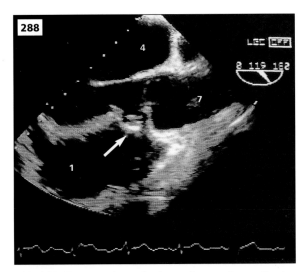

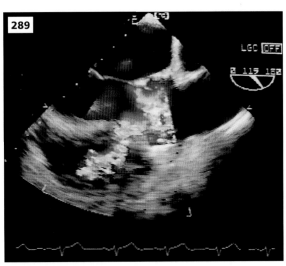

288, 289. Transesophageal echocardiogram in a patient with aortic valve disease and a ventricular septal defect, showing a vegetation on the left ventricular aspect of the ventricular septal defect where the jet of aortic regurgitation impinged upon the left ventricular wall. 1, RV; 4, LA; 7, AO.

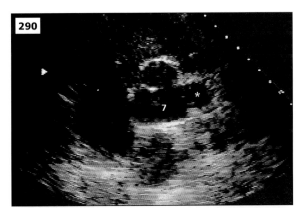

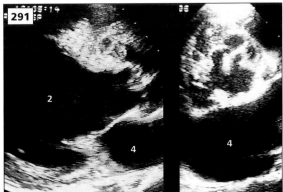

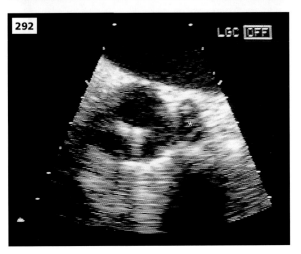

290–292. Echocardiography is essential for determining the presence of the complications of endocarditis. In particular, aortic root abscess should be examined for on a regular basis. In this example, there is a 1.5 cm rounded abscess adjacent to the left coronary cusp (*) (**290**). Mitral annular abscesses, although described, are much less common. Such abscesses may become locally invasive and this example of vegetation arising around the non- and right coronary cusps, has invaded the ventricular septum and led to complete heart block (*) (**291**). Transesophageal echocardiography may reveal small aortic root abscesses not visible by transthoracic imaging (**292**) (*). 2, LV; 4, LA; 7, AO.

Surgery is indicated in infective endocarditis for:

- Severe valvular regurgitation.
- Continuing sepsis or abscess formation.
- Emboli.

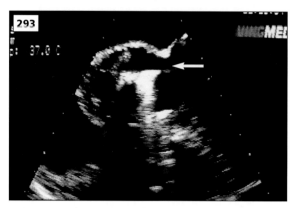

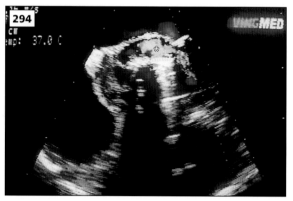

293, 294. In the presence of a prosthetic valve, localized infection may lead to dehiscence of the sewing ring. In this transesophageal example, there is a large defect in the anterior aspect of the sewing ring (arrow), with the color flow suggesting that this area is a source of regurgitation (*).

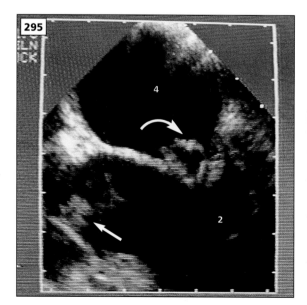

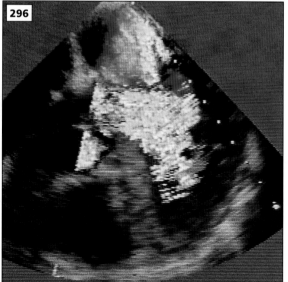

295, 296. Occasionally, infective endocarditis may affect both aortic and mitral valves. In this example, there is a large aortic vegetation shown on transesophageal imaging (straight arrow). The 1.5 cm vegetation prolapses into the left ventricular outflow tract. Note that there is left ventricular hypertrophy due to pre-existing aortic stenosis. During the course of the infective illness, mitral regurgitation occurred due to ruptured chordae tendineae with associated vegetations (curly arrow). Colour imaging confirms there is a broad jet of aortic regurgitation almost filling the left ventricle and a narrow jet of mitral regurgitation. 2, LV; 4, LA.

11 CARDIAC MASSES

While the heart may rarely be the source of primary cardiac tumors – predominantly myxomata – most tumors represent secondary involvement from extracardiac sites, particularly breast and bronchus. Differentiation of primary and secondary cardiac tumor from thrombus may be difficult.

Cardiac Tumors

Cardiac tumors are mostly due to myxomata. Less commonly found are fibroma, sarcoma, and their malignant forms (**297**). In patients with an ill-defined systemic illness, the use of echocardiography to diagnose or exclude the presence of a cardiac tumor is mandatory.

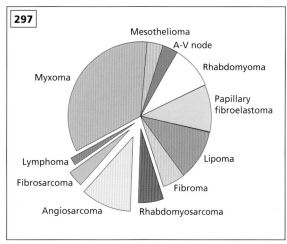

297. Incidence of cardiac tumors.

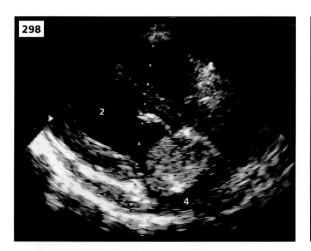

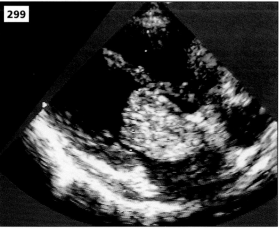

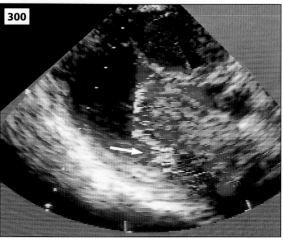

298–302. A left atrial myxoma is seen as a large heterogeneous mass lying within the atrium. It may be mobile, as in this example, where it prolapses through the mitral orifice in diastole (**299**). The size of the tumor is variable and, if sufficiently large, will cause hemodynamic obstruction. In this case, the color flow demonstrates an increase in blood velocity (arrow) round the tumor which led to a rise in left atrial pressure and mimics the signs of mitral stenosis (**300**). Short-axis views show the relationship of the tumor to the atrial septum and in this case, it appears to almost fill the atrium (**301**). The nature of the echo texture of the tumor is useful in differentiating its origin. Myxomas tend to be heterogeneous with lacunae as well as a variable amount of fibrous tissue producing dense echos; a fibrous stalk may be seen arising from the tumor, usually to the rim of the foramen ovale. The M-mode echocardiogram in this case, shows the tumor mass filling the mitral orifice in diastole (**302**). 1, RV; 2, LV; 4, LA; 7, AO.

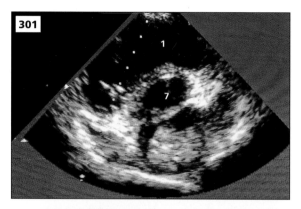

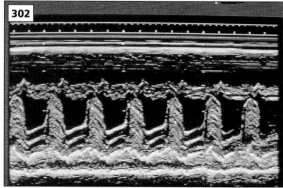

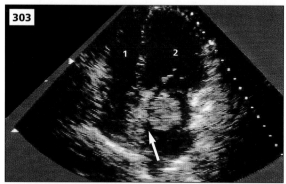

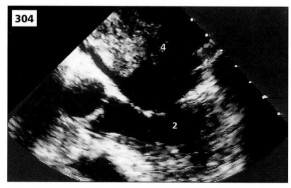

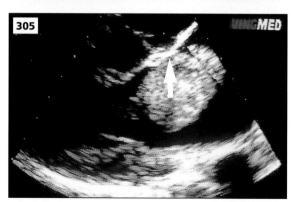

303–305. An apical four-chamber view shows the tumor attached by a pedicle which is not well-imaged but is seen as two bright echos in the area of the foramen ovale (arrow) (**303**). The nature of this mass is seen by transesophageal echocardiography (**304**). It may be useful to have epicardial imaging of the tumor during cardiac surgery to make certain that all of it is removed (**305**). In this case, the attachment, via a short pedicle to the intra-atrial septum, is well demonstrated (arrow). 1, RV; 2, LV; 4, LA.

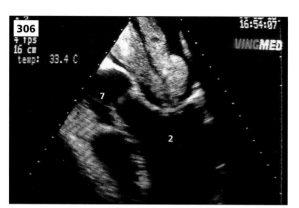

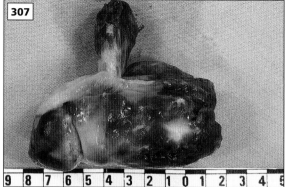

306, 307. Transesophageal echocardiography may allow the demonstration of unusual features within the myxoma. In this case, the left atrium is filled by a huge mass which is bifid. The mass appeared to move in unison and at removal of this tumor at surgery, its cleft nature was apparent. 2, LV; 7, AO.

- *Myxomas are usually obvious in that they are heterogeneous and in particular arise from a stalk from the atrial septum in the vast majority of cases.*

- *Right atrial myxomas appear to be very rare.*

- *As with all echo reporting, try not to make a diagnosis without the benefit of clinical data, as the clinical history in relation to patients with myxomas compared with thrombi may be entirely different.*

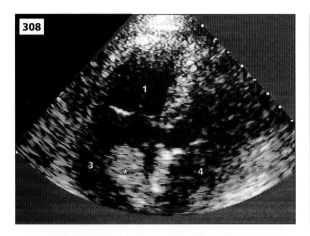

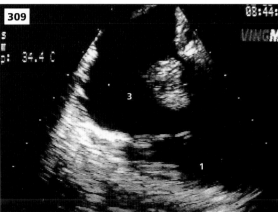

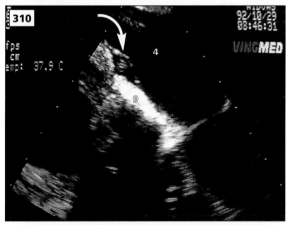

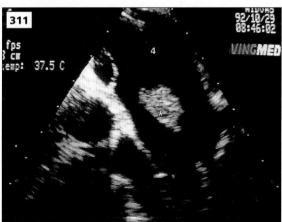

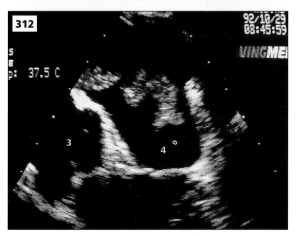

308–312. Right atrial myxomata are much less common than those in the left atrium. However, imaging of such masses is not difficult. In this case, in an apical four-chamber view, a mass is seen arising from the right side of the intra-atrial septum in the area of the foramen (*) (**308**). No definitive pedicle is seen, but the tumor has a heterogeneous appearance with lacunae within it. In such cases, transesophageal echocardiography can provide further information. In this case, the mass is seen lying within the right atrium and prolapses through the tricuspid valve in diastole (**309**). Imaging of the intra-atrial septum itself shows the mass protruding through a bulging foramen ovale (arrow) (**310**). Imaging of the left atrium shows this mass to be also present within this cavity (**311**, **312**). Even though the left atrial tumor is quite large, this was not observed by transthoracic imaging. 1, RV; 3, RA; 4, LA; 9, IAS.

Ventricular tumors

Ventricular tumors may be either intra-myocardial or intra-cavity. If there is a pericardial effusion present, it often suggests the tumor is malignant.

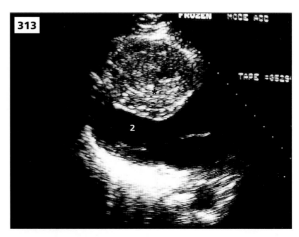

313. A tumor is shown arising in the inter-ventricular septum (*). This tumor is a low-grade malignant myoma with local invasion. Its sheer size causes hemodynamic obstruction and arrhythmias. 2, LV.

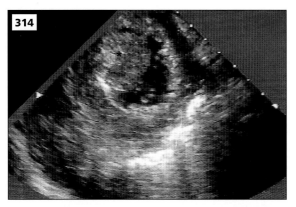

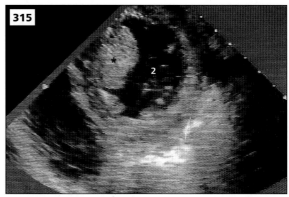

314, 315. A transgastric transesophageal view of the left ventricle in a patient with an intra-ventricular tumor. This is a large mass which arises in the ventricular septum (*).

Surprisingly, it has no effect on ventricular contraction but induced left ventricular outflow tract obstruction. 2, LV.

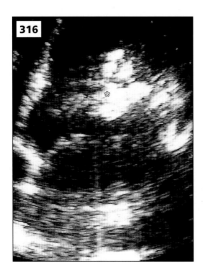

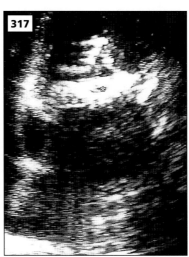

316, 317. The left ventricle may be involved by benign tumors which calcify. In this case, a fibroma is seen arising at the base of the left ventricle. There is extensive calcification (*) which masks the underlying ventricular morphology. Such tumors are very slowly progressive.

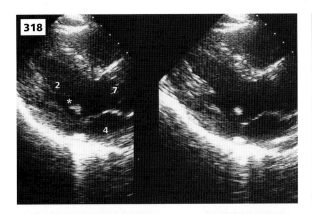

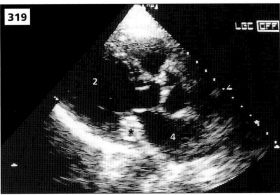

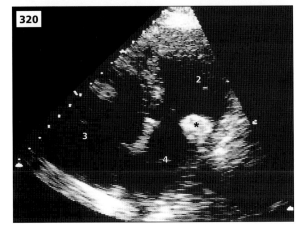

318–320. There is a variety of unusual tumors arising within the heart. Many of them, like this mitral valve papilloma (*), are associated with transient ischemic attacks (**318**). However, even large tumors of this type may be asymptomatic (**319, 320**). 2, LV; 3, RA; 4, LA; 7, AO.

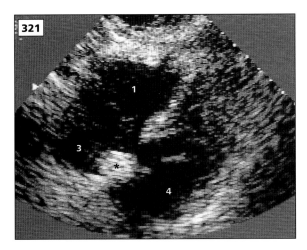

321. Atrial lipomata are relatively common, benign tumors arising in the interatrial septum (*), particularly in the elderly patient. They are rarely of any clinical consequence and are readily imaged in a sub-costal view. 1, RV; 3, RA; 4, LA.

Extracardiac Tumors

Various tumors may secondarily affect the heart. They may, as in the hypernephroma shown below (322–324), grow up the venous system into the heart. The spread of tumor may be direct, as for breast and bronchial secondaries. Occasionally, tumors may arise in the pericardium. Lymphomas may involve the myocardium directly with secondary deposits.

The heart is frequently involved in patients with widespread disseminated malignant disease and this is most frequently seen as a pericardial effusion.

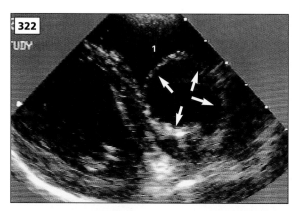

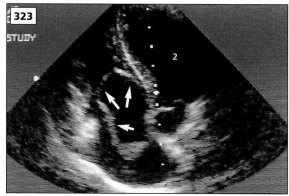

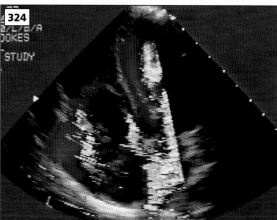

322–324. Right ventricular inlet view showing a large cystic mass prolapsing through the tricuspid valve. In an apical five-chamber view, a similar mass is seen entering the right ventricle. This was a hypernephroma involving the inferior vena cava. Color-flow imaging shows this to obstruct tricuspid inflow and it was associated with peripheral edema (**324**). 1, RV; 2, LV.

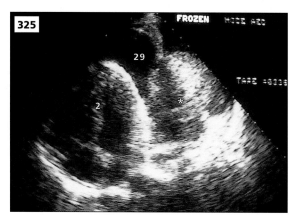

325. Lymphoma may affect the pericardium or the myocardium directly. In this case, there is a large pericardial mass (*) and pericardial effusion (29). 2, LV.

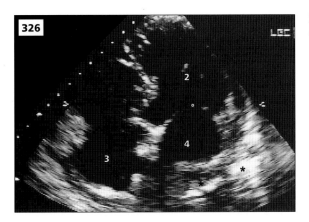

326. Esophageal tumors may envelop the heart (*). In this example the left atrium is compressed. 2, LV; 3, RA; 4, LA.

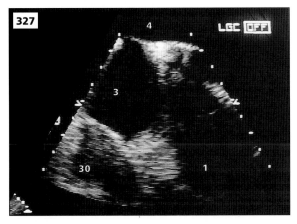

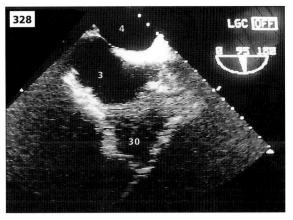

327, 328. Squamous cell carcinoma of the lung (30) invading the right atrium and inducing atrial fibrillation.

Transverse (**327**) and longitudinal (**328**) transesophageal views. 1, RV; 3, RA; 4, LA; 30, mass.

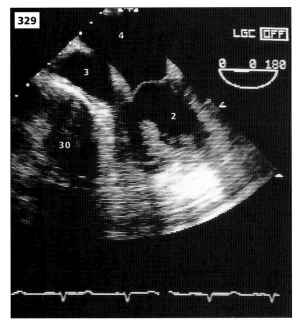

329. External compression may occur without invasion, as in this case where a large mediastinal mass (30) is seen to compress the right atrium and right ventricle on a transverse transesophageal view. 2, LV; 3, RA; 4, LA.

Intracardiac Thrombus

Intracardiac thrombus arises commonly in the left ventricle following myocardial infarction or with impaired ventricular contraction. Atrial thrombus may arise in the presence of atrial fibrillation and valvular disease. In-dwelling intravenous lines may be the source of thrombus formation.

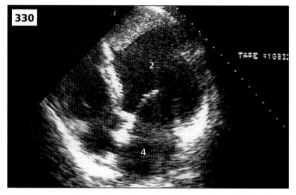

330. An apical four-chamber view in a patient following myocardial infarction. There is a large adherent (laminated) stable ventricular thrombus (*). In contrast to a myxoma, this has a homogeneous appearance and the mass arises in an area of dyskinesis. 2, LV; 4, LA.

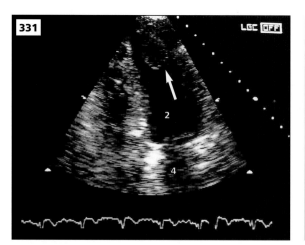

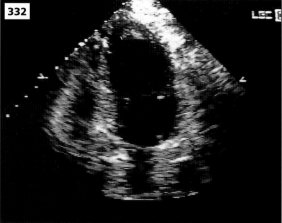

331, 332. Pair of apical four-chamber views showing a pedunculated thrombus with an echolucent center (arrow). This type of thrombus may be unstable and is seen to have embolized to the leg on the following day. 2, LV; 4, LA.

- *In many patients it may be difficult to obtain high-quality images of the ventricular apex. In addition there may be artifacts which obscure this area, or suggest the presence of apical thrombus. If there is doubt, it is useful to assess regional contraction as thrombus only arises in areas of myocardial damage.*

- *Intracardiac thrombus needs to have a cause and if abnormal echos suggest its presence in an otherwise normal heart, the diagnosis must be reconsidered.*

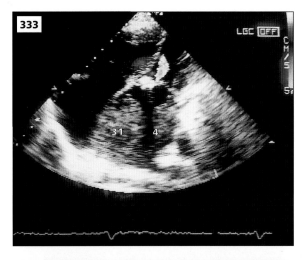

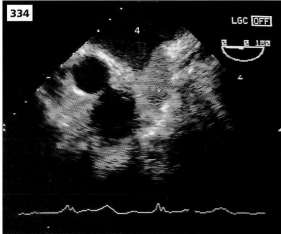

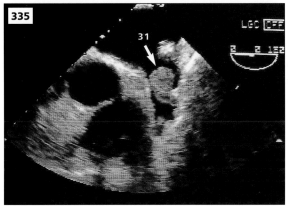

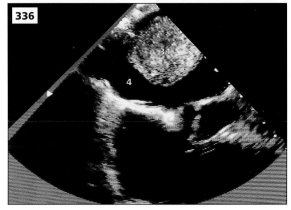

333–336. Left atrial thrombus is common in mitral stenosis. Occasionally, the thrombus (31) may be seen adherent to the septum and posterior atrial wall (**333**). However, transesophageal echocardiography allows imaging of the left atrial appendage. In this example the appendage is filled with a mobile thrombus (*) (**334**). The thrombus can be more discrete (**335**) or enlarge to form a ball valve (**336**). 4, LA; 31, thrombus.

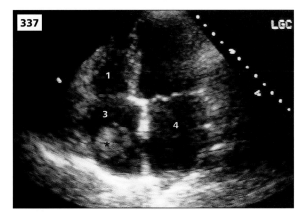

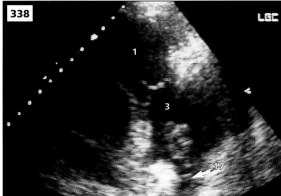

337–343. Thrombus may arise in the right atrium, either *de novo*, or extend from the venous system. **337** shows a rounded mass in the right atrium (*) which is difficult to differentiate from a myxoma, but by the right atrial inlet view it can be seen to extend from the inferior vena cava, suggesting a thrombotic origin (**338**). The appearance of thrombus may suggest its origin. In a man with postoperative pulmonary embolism, transesophageal echocardiography revealed a serpiginous mobile thrombus resembling a venous cast (arrow). (*Cont.*) 1, RV; 3, RA; 4, LA; 17, IVC.

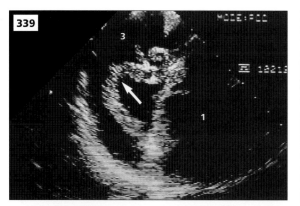

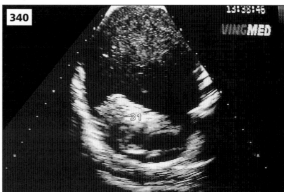

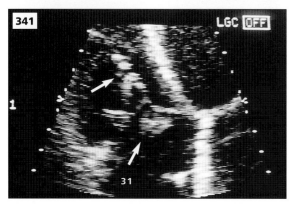

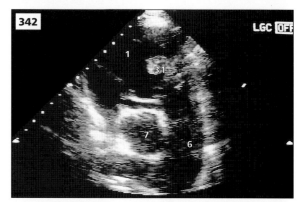

337–343. (*Cont.*) The thrombus in **338** was seen to extend into the right ventricle and pulmonary artery (**339**, arrow). In long-standing tricuspid valve disease – in this case a stenosed tricuspid valve replacement – sessile calcified thrombus (31) is seen with 'smoke' in a huge right atrium by transesophageal imaging (**340**). Thrombus may arise at the site of intracardiac in-dwelling lines and lead occasionally to embolization. Transthoracic imaging shows thrombus (31) associated with a permanent right ventricular pacing electrode (**341**). Pacing wires often look thicker than they are because of internal reverberations and motion artifact, but in this case thrombus (31) is seen on the right atrial aspect of the tricuspid valve. Long-standing pulmonary artery catheters may result in thrombus (31) in the right ventricular outflow tract (**342**). Less commonly, cerebral shunts terminating in the right atrium may lead to thrombus (31) formation – in this case with embolization and pulmonary hypertension (**343**). 1, RV; 3, RA; 6, PA; 7, AO.

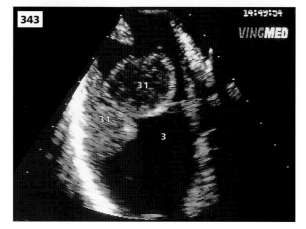

12 PERICARDIAL DISEASE

Pericardial fluid may be readily demonstrated by cardiac ultrasound. With improving technology, small amounts of fluid may be seen, even in normal individuals. The presence of pericardial fluid may be a useful diagnostic feature in a variety of diseases.

An approximate guide to a pericardial effusion may be made by measuring the depth of effusion.

- *Small <1 cm.*
- *Moderate 1–2 cm.*
- *Large >2 cm.*

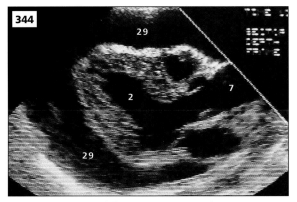

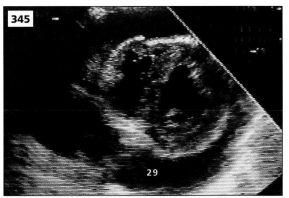

344, 345. Long- and short-axis parasternal views in a patient with a large pericardial effusion (29). This is shown both anteriorly and posteriorly. The heart moves or swings markedly during the cardiac cycle. 2, LV; 7, AO.

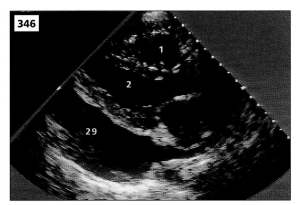

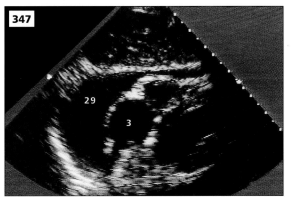

346, 347. The effusion may be unevenly distributed and therefore it is important to image from all possible windows. In this case, a large posterior effusion is seen with an otherwise normal heart. By subcostal views, the inferior surface of the heart has only a small effusion, though it is much larger overlying the right atrium.

M-mode echocardiography does demonstrate the presence of effusions, though is relatively unhelpful. It is very difficult to assess ventricular function in the presence of pericardial effusion (29) because of the movement of the heart within the M-mode beam. 1, RV; 2, LV; 3, RA.

The rate of accumulation of pericardial fluid is an important factor in the consequent hemodynamic effects of the effusion.

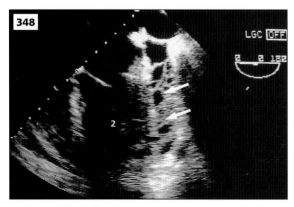

348. Fibrin strands (arrows) within the pericardial effusion. This feature may be useful in the diagnosis of infective pericarditis, though is also seen in patients with malignant and hemorrhagic effusions. 2, LV.

Tips to help distinguish pleural from pericardial fluid:

- *Clinical examination and chest radiograph may suggest pleural fluid.*
- *The position of the descending aorta on the parasternal long axis view is useful. Large pericardial effusions typically expand behind the left atrium, displacing the extrapericardial aorta posteriorly. A pleural effusion remains posterior to the descending aorta.*
- *There may be the characteristic appearance of collapsed lung tissue within a pleural effusion.*
- *A large amount of fluid without 'bobbing' of the heart or signs of tamponade favor a pleural effusion.*
- *Fluid between the diaphragm and heart in the subcostal view is always pericardial.*

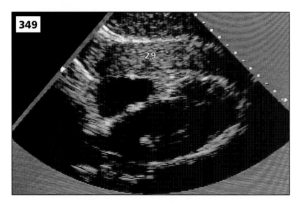

349. Cardiac tamponade is difficult to diagnose with certainty by echocardiography. Such diagnosis is probably best made clinically with examination of the venous pressure, peripheral pulse, and blood pressure. There may be some useful echocardiographic indicators to this diagnosis. Firstly, a diagnosis of pericardial effusion, secondly exaggerated movement of the heart within this effusion, and thirdly diastolic collapse of the right ventricle. Although these are useful features none of them is pathognomonic. Doppler studies demonstrate exaggerated respiratory variation in blood flow through the right and left heart. In this example, shown by subcostal views, there is a large pericardial effusion (29) which is homogeneous in appearance due to postoperative hemorrhage with subsequent clotting.

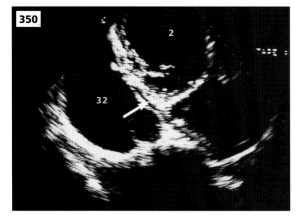

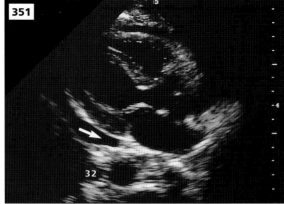

350, 351. It may be difficult to differentiate pleural from pericardial fluid. In most cases of pleural effusion of a respiratory origin there is no associated pericardial fluid. However, in patients with heart failure, the pleural effusion (32) is often associated with a small pericardial effusion (arrow) and differentiation is seen clearly in these examples. 2, LV.

Pericardial constriction, both acute and chronic, is rare in the West. The chronic forms are mostly due to previous tuberculous and viral infections. Following viral infection, many patients have a thickened pericardium which is not constrictive but may become so (352).

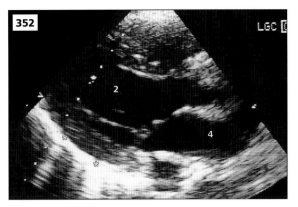

352. Thickened pericardium (*) following viral infection, which is not constrictive but may become so. 2, LV; 4, LA.

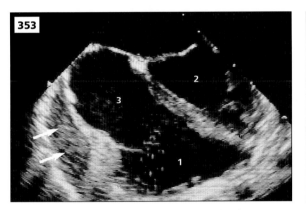

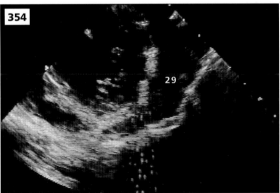

353, 354. Transesophageal echocardiography shows a patient with acute tuberculous pericarditis associated with pulmonary disease. The pericardium overlying the right atrioventricular (AV) groove is enormously thickened without obvious fluid (arrows). However, over the left AV groove there is a pericardial effusion (29). This patient had hemodynamic evidence of constriction and underwent a pericardial resection. 1, RV; 2, LV; 3, RA.

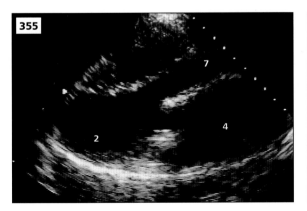

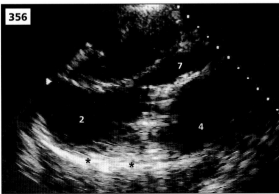

355, 356. Chronic constrictive pericarditis is much more difficult to image as a thickened pericardium with calcification leads to echo-masking. However, in this patient with a mitral prosthesis there is thickening and calcification of the posterior pericardium (*). 2, LC; 4, LA; 7, Aorta.

- *The pericardium often looks 'bright' on phased array echo systems by the nature of their post-processing.*
- *As the resolution of echo systems has improved it is apparent that many normal studies have a pericardial effusion.*

357. In this parasternal long-axis view the pericardium posterior to the left ventricle is thickened and calcified (*). While imaging in real-time the left ventricle appeared tethered to the pericardium at this site. 2, LV; 4, LA.

The movement of the left ventricle in pericardial constriction is quite abnormal. It has a jerky incoordinate appearance, but overall contraction may be normal. It is important to differentiate constrictive pericarditis from restricted cardiomyopathy. This is best dealt with by the demonstration of the constellation of physical findings, imaging of the pericardium and myocardium, and Doppler traces.

Echocardiographic features of pericardial constriction include:

- *Thickened pericardium (normal approximately 4 mm). This may be better assessed by CT or MRI scanning.*
- *M-mode may demonstrate early cessation of diastolic filling (often referred to as left ventricular posterior wall 'flattening') and shortened deceleration time.*
- *Left ventricular motion may be 'jerky' due to abnormal filling.*
- *There may be a septal 'bounce'.*
- *Marked inspiratory fall in peak mitral E-wave velocity.*
- *Reciprocal changes in tricuspid flow velocity with increased velocity on inspiration.*
- *Shortening of mitral and tricuspid valve deceleration times.*
- *Exaggerated flow reversal in the SVC on expiration.*

If the diagnosis is in doubt then cardiac catheterization may be performed and demonstrates equal end-diastolic pressures in all four chambers.

13 THORACIC AORTIC DISSECTION

The terminology used to classify aortic dissection may be confusing as there are two classification systems in use (358). The site of entry tear and proximal extension determine the type of dissection. The Stanford classification simply divides dissections into those involving the ascending aorta (Type A) and those that spare it (Type B). This has the advantage of identifying those dissections in which operation is indicated (A) and those in whom conservative treatment is preferred (B). DeBakey classifies dissections into three types:

Type I involves ascending and descending aorta (Stanford A)

Type II involves only the ascending aorta (Stanford A)

Type III involves the descending aorta (Stanford B)

The development of transesophageal echocardiography has revolutionized the management of patients with aortic disease. It is now the diagnostic method of choice for dissection and exceeds CT scanning in specificity and sensitivity, and equals that of magnetic resonance imaging. Of course, it has the advantage of being able to be undertaken in an anesthetic room or intensive care unit, in contrast to the need for the patient to lie flat in an imaging department. The imaging of dissection flaps and thrombus is relatively straightforward and they are usually readily seen. Recently, transesophageal imaging of aortic atheromatous plaques has proved important in the diagnosis of emboli.

Clinical features of aortic dissection include:

- *Chest pain – severe, often 'tearing' and may radiate to the back.*
- *Possible history of hypertension or collagen vascular abnormalities.*
- *Aortic regurgitation.*
- *Asymmetric pulses.*
- *Difference in systolic blood pressure between right and left arms of >25 mmHg.*
- *There may be neurologic signs.*
- *Chest radiograph may demonstrate widened mediastinum.*

Echocardiography in aortic dissection aims to diagnose:

- *Presence of aortic dissection.*
- *Involvement of ascending aorta and extent of dissection.*
- *Entry sites.*
- *Aortic valve function.*
- *Proximal coronary artery involvement.*
- *Branch vessel involvement.*
- *Left ventricular function.*
- *Pericardial effusion.*

358	DeBakey	
Type I Proximal tear. Dissection involves ascending and descending aorta	**Type II** Proximal tear. Dissection confined to ascending aorta	**Type III** Tear beyond subclavian. Dissection confined to descending aorta
Type A Dissection involves ascending aorta with or without descending aorta		**Type B** Dissection confined to descending aorta
Stanford		

358. The classification of aortic dissection.

Table 14 shows a comparison of imaging techniques for the evaluation of suspected aortic dissection.

Table 14. Imaging techniques and evaluation of aortic dissection	TEE	CT	MRI	Aortography
Sensitivity	+++	++	+++	++
Specificity	++/+++	+++	+++	+++
Entry tears	++	+	+++	++
Aortic regurgitation	+++	–	+	+++
Coronary arteries	++	–	+	++
Branch vessels	+	+	++	+++
Pericardial effusion	+++	++	+++	–
Convenience	+++	++	+	+

359. Long-axis transesophageal view of an aneurysmal ascending aorta with dissection (33). The aortic valve is thickened but unobstructive (arrow).

- Because echocardiography, including transesophageal study, can be performed at the bedside this should be the initial investigation in centers with transthoracic echocardiography expertise.

- As an ascending aortic dissection flap may be seen by transthoracic echocardiography, we recommend a transthoracic scan first. If a Type A dissection is diagnosed we then perform a transesophageal echocardiography in the anesthetic room peri-operatively with the patient anesthetized and monitored.

Risk factors for aortic dissection include hypertension, connective tissue diseases (particularly Marfan's syndrome), coarctation of the aorta and pregnancy.

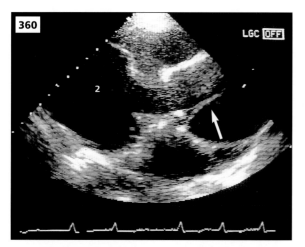

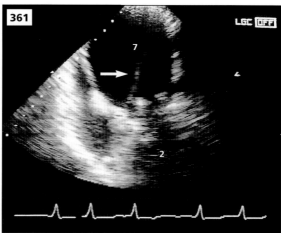

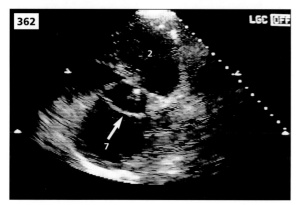

360–362. Transthoracic echocardiography may occasionally image ascending aortic dissections. By a parasternal long-axis view there is an intimal flap arising (arrow) just above the valve in a dilated ascending aorta (**360**). By a modified right parasternal window the flap is seen extending into the ascending aorta (**361**). It is important to image all available windows and in this case only the five-chambered view showed an ascending flap (**362**). If the transthoracic echocardiogram diagnoses an ascending aortic dissection the patient may be transferred to the operating room for a peri-operative/intra-operative transesophageal echocardiogram without delay. 2, LV; 7, AO.

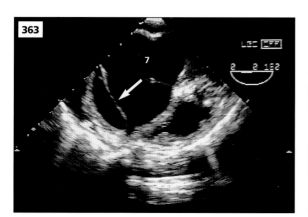

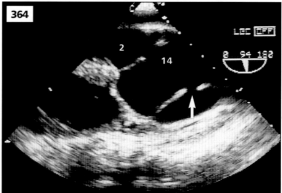

363, 364. An ascending aortic dissection is seen by transesophageal echo as a flap lying above the aortic valve (**363**, arrow). Imaging in the long axis shows the aorta to be grossly dilated with an intimal tear (**364**, arrow). 2, LV; 7, AO; 14, AoV.

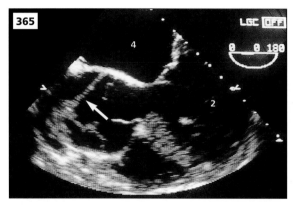

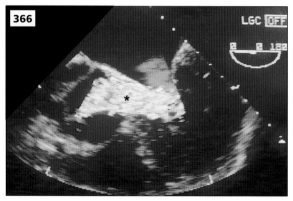

365, 366. The intimal flap (arrow) is usually seen in motion during the cardiac cycle. In this case it arises just above the aortic valve and disrupts its function. Color flow shows there to be a regurgitant jet (*). 2, LV; 4, LA.

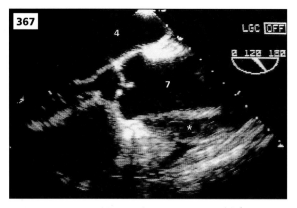

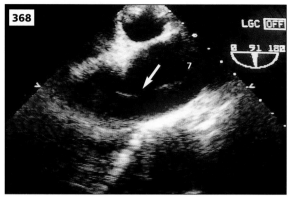

367. In a patient with a clinical syndrome suggestive of dissection, transesophageal echo may not show a dissection flap but localized intramural hemorrhage (*) which leads to cardiac tamponade. 4, LA; 7, AO.

368. Artifact from the aortic wall may produce an echo-dense linear structure within the ascending aorta (arrow) which must be differentiated from a dissection flap. 7, AO.

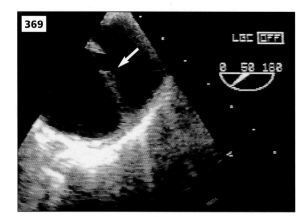

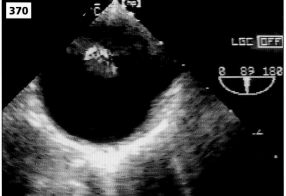

369, 370. The site of dissection tear may be in the arch rather than the ascending aorta (the proximal arch remains difficult to image because of the position of the trachea). However, in the distal arch the dissection flaps are readily seen by transesophageal echo (arrow) and flow between the true to false lumen may be seen by color flow (**370**).

Errors in the diagnosis of aortic dissection by transesophageal echocardiography are usually due to reverberation artifacts in the ascending aorta. Artifact is usually linear and parallel to the aortic wall. It has a fixed relationship to the aorta without

independent motion, unlike dissection flaps which are usually obvious and, unless thrombosed, move with the cardiac cycle. In addition, true intimal flaps should be visible in more than one plane.

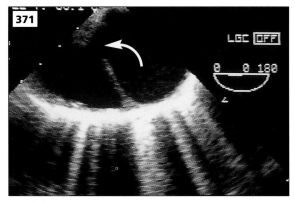

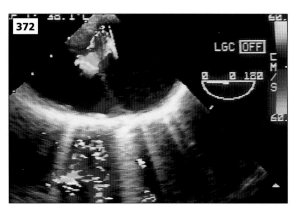

371, 372. An entry tear is clearly seen in the distal arch (**371**, arrow) with color flow from true to false lumen (**372**).

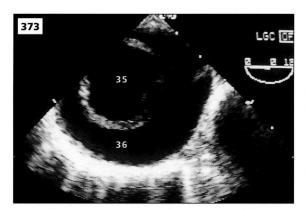

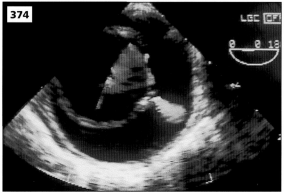

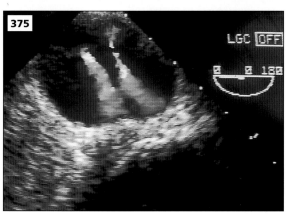

373–375. The descending aorta is readily imaged by transthoracic or transesophageal echocardiography. In this example the true lumen (35) is surrounded by a false lumen (36) and flow is seen between them by color-flow Doppler (**374**). The blood flow within the false lumen is often slow and thrombus formation may occur; it may also be difficult to differentiate between the false and true lumen. The false lumen tends not to give rise to main vessels and the flow tends to be slow, or delayed, within the lumen body. The true lumen tends to have systolic expansion, and color-flow jets may be seen passing from true to false lumen. Occasionally, multiple tear sites are demonstrated (**375**).

The true lumen may be smaller than the false lumen. The true lumen expands in systole.

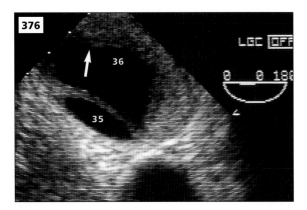

376. A dissection flap is seen within the descending aorta. The false lumen (36) is large and partially filled with thrombus (arrow). True lumen (35) can also be seen.

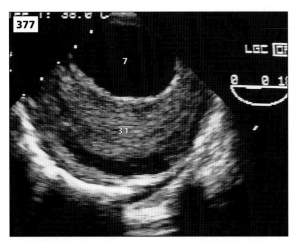

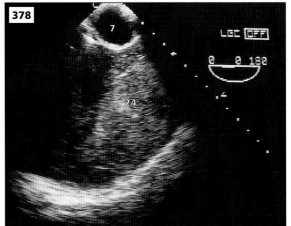

377, 378. True aneurysms of the descending aorta may be large and often filled with thrombus (31) (**377**); in addition, extensive hematoma (24) may be seen occasionally around the aorta (**378**). 7, AO.

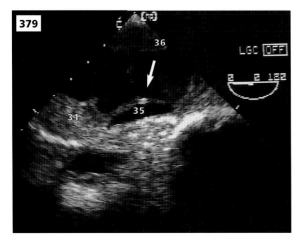

379. In this example a dissection has occurred in an aneurysmal descending aorta. The intimal flap is readily appreciated (arrow) and the aneurysm has considerable thrombus (31) within. Both the true lumen (35) and the false lumen (36) can be seen.

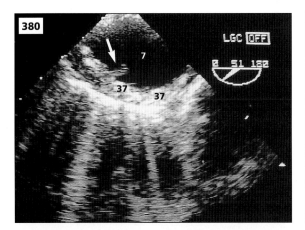

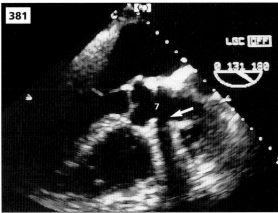

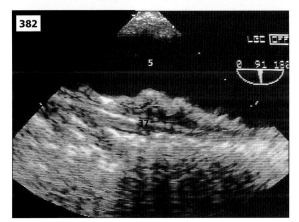

380–382. Atheroma in the ascending aorta may be the site of cerebral emboli, especially if they are large with associated thrombus (arrow) (**380**). However, even small calcified plaques (in this case seen with acoustic shadowing) may be important (arrow) (**381**). Plaque (37) may also be demonstrated in the descending aorta (**382**). 5, DAO; 7, AO.

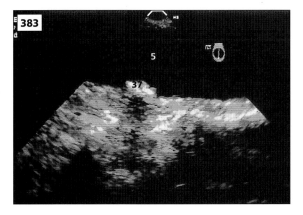

383. This demonstrates a calcified plaque (37) in the descending aorta with acoustic shadowing imaged in the long-axis view. 5, DAO.

Mural hematoma may herald an acute dissection and should be treated in the same way as aortic dissection.

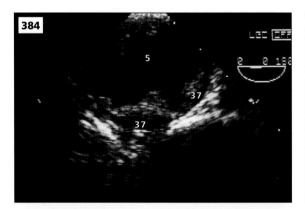

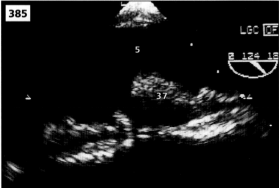

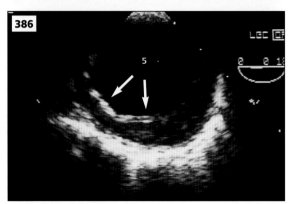

384–386. Atheroma may be very extensive – as in this example, where there are large, irregular craggy heaps of atheroma (**384, 385**). The long-axis view (**385**) shows a protuberation of atheroma (37) into the lumen of the descending aorta. Atheroma is often irregular; this helps differentiate it from thrombus, which usually has a layered or laminated appearance (arrow) (**386**). Atheroma may of course be associated with overlying thrombus formation. 5, DAO.

14 CORONARY ARTERY DISEASE

Echocardiography may be used to study patients with coronary artery disease in a number of ways. Unfortunately, standard transthoracic and transesophageal echocardiography reveal little of the coronary tree that is of clinical relevance. In the acute phase, impairment of left ventricular contraction, thrombus formation, aneurysm, ventricular septal rupture, and mitral regurgitation may all be demonstrated. In the chronic phase, thrombus formation, aneurysm, and impaired left ventricular contraction may also be observed. Stress echocardiography may be used as a substitute for perfusion scanning to determine areas of regional wall motion abnormality in ischemia and also viable myocardium. Coronary arteries may be imaged directly and intra-arterial probes may give unique views of the coronary anatomy.

Echocardiography is invaluable in the coronary care unit. It may be argued that in a busy unit with a large throughput of patients, an echo machine should be permanently available. Of particular use is the diagnosis of non-coronary causes of chest pain and the examination of patients with murmurs and heart failure.

Acute Myocardial Infarction

The echocardiogram may be valuable in examining patients who have recently suffered a myocardial infarction. The most common finding would be an area of regional wall motion abnormality with reduced contraction and delayed relaxation. In the early phases of myocardial infarction, the myocardium is not thinned and the ventricular cavity is of normal size. Ventricular dilatation and compensatory hypertrophy of the non-infarcted segments does not occur for some weeks or months. Following a myocardial infarction, there may be intracavity ventricular thrombus. This more commonly occurs following anterior infarctions and therefore is antero-apical in site. Examination of the acute complications of myocardial infarction, such as mitral regurgitation, ventricular septal rupture, and ventricular rupture and tamponade, can all be observed by echocardiography. The echocardiogram may be particularly helpful in the differential diagnosis of a patient complaining of chest pain with an abnormal electrocardiogram. This differential diagnosis may include hypertrophic cardiomyopathy, aortic valve disease, and other structural cardiac disorders without ischemia.

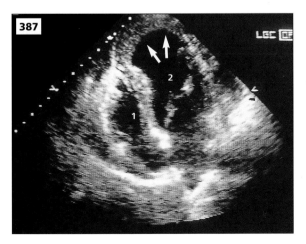

387. Apical four-chamber view in a patient who has recently suffered a myocardial infarction. There is an area of apical thrombus which has a homogeneous appearance (arrows). The base of the left ventricle is slightly dilated and if examined during the cardiac cycle the apex is seen to be akinetic. If there is difficulty with a differential diagnosis of an area at the apex, a useful rule is that thrombus only overlies akinetic areas. 1, RV; 2, LV.

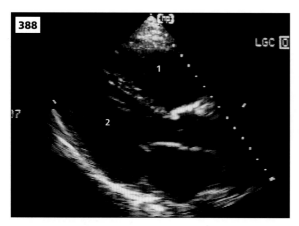

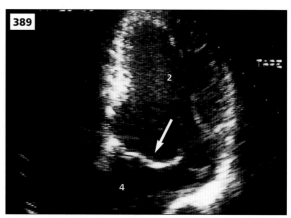

388. Right ventricular infarcts occur in approximately 25% of inferior infarcts and are clinically significant in 10%. The clinical signs include a greatly elevated jugular venous pressure, hypotension, and clear lung fields. The right ventricle is dilated and impaired on echo, as shown on this long-axis parasternal view. 1, RV; 2, LV

389. Apical four-chamber view showing prolapse of the posterior leaflet of the mitral valve (arrow). This is a patient who has suffered a localized inferior infarction affecting predominantly the posterolateral papillary muscle. There is acute mitral regurgitation which requires urgent surgical intervention. Quite frequently the patient presenting with mitral regurgitation post-myocardial infarction has limited myocardial damage. 2, LV; 4, LA.

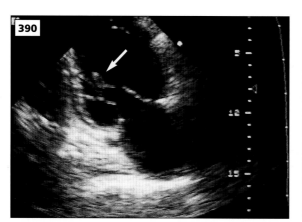

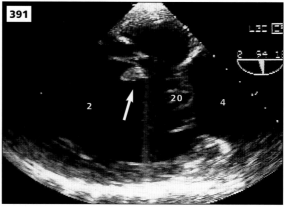

390, 391. Occasionally, papillary muscle rupture may occur with gross mitral regurgitation. The posterior papillary muscle (arrow) is seen avulsed and moving with the flail mitral valve by both transthoracic (**390**) and transesophageal (transgastric longitudinal view) (**391**) echocardiography. 2, LV; 4, LA; 20, MV.

- *Post-infarction ventricular septal defects may only be evident on angling the transducer superiorly or inferiorly from standard four-chamber views.*

- *VSDs only occur in infarcted walls; therefore, if there is suspicious color flow, but the underlying ventricular function is normal, another diagnosis must be considered.*

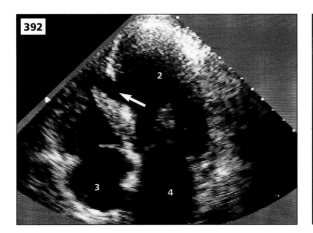

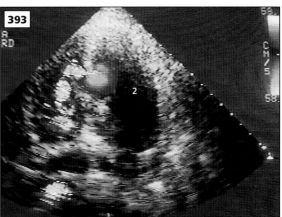

392, 393. The other cause of an acute development of a systolic murmur post-myocardial infarction is ventricular septal rupture. This occurs due to hemorrhage into the myocardium of the septum with subsequent rupturing into the right ventricle. The echocardiographic appearances of this are usually readily apparent. In particular, the area of a ventricular septum is akinetic and often has an unusual appearance where the two edges do not seem to align. In this apical four-chamber view, the misalignment of the septum is quite clearly seen (arrow) (**392**). There is a color flow jet through this representing a left-to-right shunt (**393**). The movement of the ventricular septum is also abnormal because the myocardium around the defect is akinetic and there may be hyperdynamic contraction in the other portions. As the severity of left-to-right shunting progresses, right ventricular size increases and contraction becomes impaired, which is a poor prognostic feature. 2, LV; 3, RA; 4, LA.

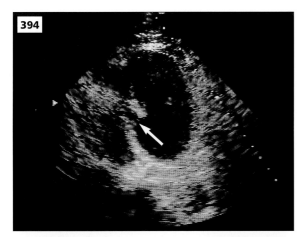

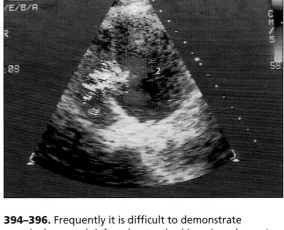

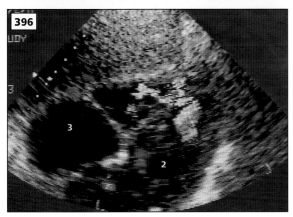

394–396. Frequently it is difficult to demonstrate ventricular septal defects by standard imaging planes. In this case, a superior angulated four-chamber view is needed to show the misalignment of the ventricular septum (arrow) (**394**). A broad jet of color flow is shown across this defect (**395**). Similarly, it may be necessary to use subcostal imaging to demonstrate a ventricular septal defect. The defect is towards the apex which makes it more difficult to image (**396**). There is a flow pattern across the ventricular septum with high velocity on the left ventricular aspect due to flow convergence. 2, LV; 3, RA.

Chronic Coronary Artery Disease

In a patient with chronic coronary artery disease, the left ventricle may appear normal, or there may be areas of regional wall motion abnormality. Aneurysms and thrombi may be seen and reversible impairment of regional contraction may be demonstrated by stress echocardiography.

In ischemic heart disease where there is a regional wall motion abnormality, a wall motion score index (see 'Stress echocardiography', p. 116) may be the most accurate assessment of ejection fraction. M-mode measurements of wall thickness are taken through the basal septum and posterior walls, and can only reflect global left ventricular function if there are no regional wall motion abnormalities. Similarly, planimetry of the endocardial border assessed on both apical four-chamber and two-chamber views is satisfactory when left ventricular impairment is global, but not in coronary artery disease as regional wall motion abnormalities are too complex to be described in only two views.

Pseudoaneurysms occur after subacute rupture. These are differentiated from true aneurysms by having a narrow neck and require urgent surgery.

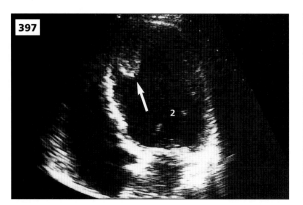

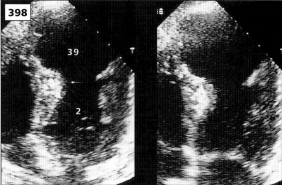

397. An apical four-chamber view showing a 'finger-like' ventricular thrombus arising from the apex (arrow). This patient suffered an extensive apical infarct with akinesis of the apex and free wall. These long, non-laminated thrombi are often of recent origin and give rise to emboli. In this case, this thrombus was seen to have partly embolized following a cerebral vascular accident. 2, LV.

398. Systolic and diastolic frames in a patient who has an extensive apical infarct. In this chronic example, there is compensatory hypertrophy with normal left ventricular contraction at the base of the heart. Dilatation at the base of the left ventricle is a poor prognostic feature for survival following surgery. 2, LV; 39, Aneurysm.

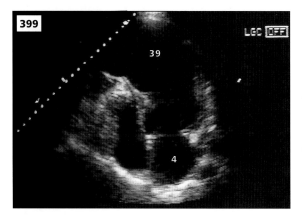

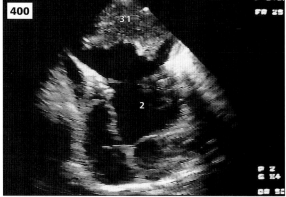

399, 400. Transthoracic echocardiography may demonstrate an apical aneurysm (39), but it is difficult to confirm paradoxical wall motion. Frequently, the

aneurysmal sac contains laminated thrombus (31) (**400**). 2, LV; 4, LA.

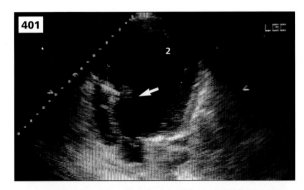

401. In this example a large antero-apical aneurysm is lined with laminated thrombus, but a small mobile thrombus (arrow) is also present. 2, LV.

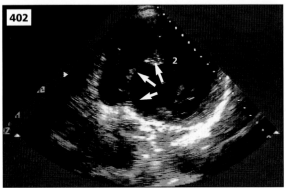

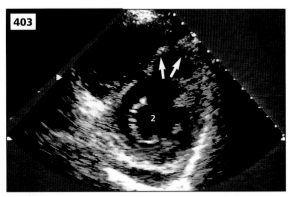

402, 403. While it is most common to have apical aneurysms, they may also occur around the base of the left ventricle. In these two examples, aneurysms of the upper portion of the septum are seen. In a modified apical four-chamber view, a discrete, thinned aneurysmal dilatation adjacent to the mitral annulus is shown (arrows). Parasternal short-axis view showing a discrete anterior ventricular aneurysm which could lead to right ventricular outflow tract obstruction (arrows) (**403**). 2, LV.

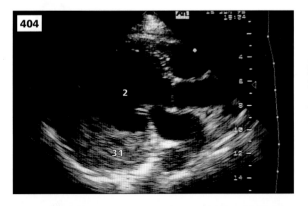

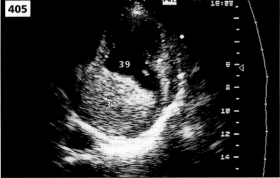

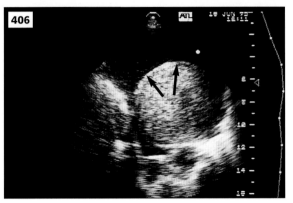

404–406. These parasternal long-axis views show a large posterior aneurysm (39) with thrombus within (31) (**404**). Angulation from an apical long-axis image shows the extent of the aneurysm (**405**). Further posterior angulation emphasizes the thin wall of the aneurysm (arrows) (**406**). 2, LV.

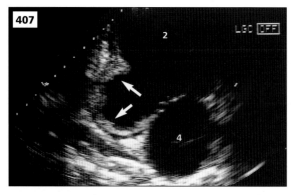

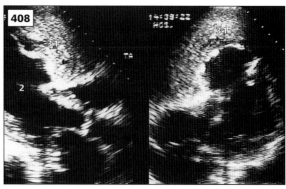

407. Apical two-chamber image demonstrating a large inferior left ventricular aneurysm (arrows) with a thin layer of laminated thrombus. The wide neck of this true aneurysm is apparent. 2, LV; 4, LA.

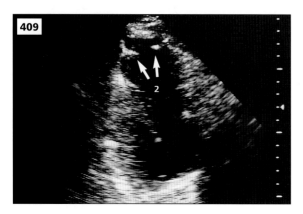

408. Occasionally, following subacute ventricular rupture, there may be the formation of a false aneurysm. These are readily differentiated from true aneurysms by their size and site, but also have a narrow neck and there is intact myocardium around the defect. They are often extensively filled with thrombus. In this example, in apical two-chamber and subcostal views, a huge defect is shown anteriorly which is filled with thrombus (31). There is, in addition, a dyskinetic area around the defect of the rupture and this represents a true aneurysm of the ventricular septum. 2, LV.

409. Apical recording of a small apical pseudo-aneurysm with a narrow neck (arrows). 2, LV.

Left Ventricular Function in Coronary Heart Disease

Left ventricular contraction in coronary heart disease is differentiated from most other forms of heart disease by its regional or dyskinetic nature.

Occasionally, it may be difficult to differentiate apical hypertrophy, especially with muscle bands present, from thrombus. If apical contraction is normal, the likelihood of thrombus is extremely low.

Stress echocardiography

Stress echocardiography combines cross-sectional imaging with an ischemic stressor. Although exercise is the best stressor for induction of myocardial ischemia, from a practical point of view it is easier to obtain adequate echocardiographic images using pharmacologic stress, either with dobutamine or, less commonly, vasodilators such as dipyridamole or adenosine.

Indications for stress echocardiography include:

- *Diagnosis of coronary artery disease:*
  - *exercise test non-diagnostic or equivocal, unable to exercise*
  - *electrocardiography precludes adequate interpretation (left bundle branch block, digoxin effect, hypertension).*
- *Assessment of functional effects of coronary stenoses.*
- *Risk stratification after myocardial infarction.*
- *Assessment of myocardial viability.*

The technique is based on detecting a regional wall motion abnormality elicited by stress. As the myocardium becomes ischemic abnormalities in wall motion precede symptoms and electrocardiographic changes. The normal response to stress is hyperkinesis, increased myocardial thickening, and an increased ejection fraction. Response to stress is evaluated using a wall motion scoring index according to the system suggested by the American Society of Echocardiography (**410**), applied to a 16-segment wall model: Score 1, normal; 2, hypokinetic; 3, akinetic; 4, dyskinetic. An abnormal response is failure to develop hyperkinesis or deterioration in wall motion (hypokinesis or akinesis). In order to facilitate recognition of wall motion abnormalities, stress echo packages use a quad-screen format to display views taken at different times side-by-side. Using a dobutamine stress protocol the standard format is to display rest, low dose, peak stress and recovery on the quad screen format for each echo plane imaged. In practice, the echo planes used are the long-axis parasternal, short-axis parasternal, apical four-chamber and apical two-chamber as all wall segments and coronary territories are imaged using these views (**410**). Dedicated stress echo packages may also include software which allows overlay of color coding of systolic motion to improve the qualitative assessment of wall contractility. The number of segments affected, the degree of deterioration in wall motion and the time to onset of abnormalities help in the evaluation of the severity of the underlying coronary artery disease.

Stress echocardiography is superior to exercise *electro*cardiography for the detection of coronary artery disease and has a similar sensitivity and specificity to thallium or sesta MIBI scanning with the advantage of wide availability, low cost and avoidance of ionizing radiation.

Dobutamine stress echocardiography may also be used to detect myocardial viability. In severely impaired ventricles apparently akinetic segments of ventricle may be hibernating. If blood supply to these segments is improved, as with revascularization, then this muscle may resume normal function. Viable myocardium is identified by improvement in contraction at low-dose dobutamine with impairment of function at higher doses.

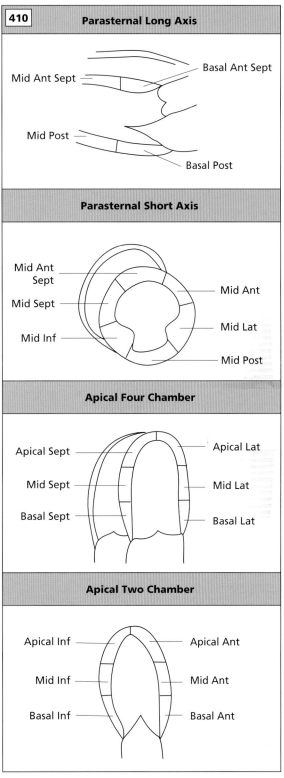

410. American Society of Echocardiography wall motion scoring index to evaluate response to stress: Score: 1, normal; 2, hypokinetic; 3, akinetic; 4, dyskinetic. These scores are applied to the 16-segment wall model illustrated.

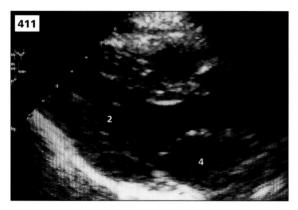

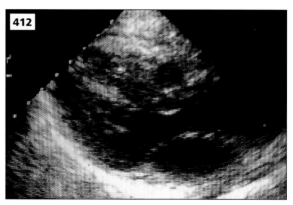

411, 412. This parasternal long-axis view demonstrates the response to stress in the normal heart. Both the anterior-septum and posterior walls become hyperkinetic

(**412**) with increased myocardial work compared with the resting image (**411**). 2, LV; 4, LA.

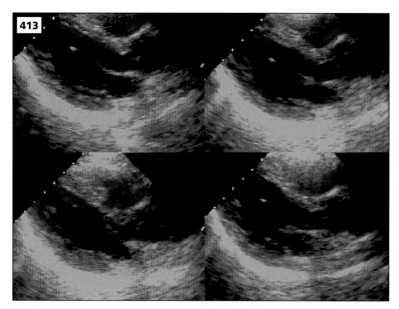

413. A quad screen format [same patient as (**411**)] of the parasternal long-axis view with color overlay to enhance motion analysis. The top left-hand image is at rest, the top right at low-dose dobutamine, the bottom left at peak stress, and the bottom right is taken during recovery. Background diastole is colored in light blue and systolic motion in red. Color enhancement 'draws' the eye to systolic events and may improve qualitative evaluation of wall motion. This example is a normal response to stress with increased systolic motion at peak stress clearly evident.

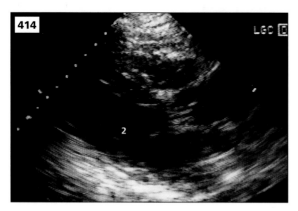

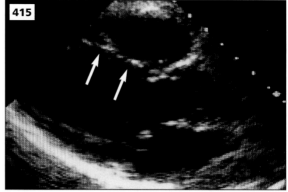

414, 415. This patient, who had a previous posterior infarct, continued to have atypical chest pain. At rest, the anteroseptum is seen to thicken normally, although the posterior wall is thin. During dobutamine stress the

posterior wall remained unchanged but the anterior septum becomes thin and akinetic (arrows). Subsequent coronary angiography demonstrated a significant stenosis in the left anterior descending coronary artery. 2, LV.

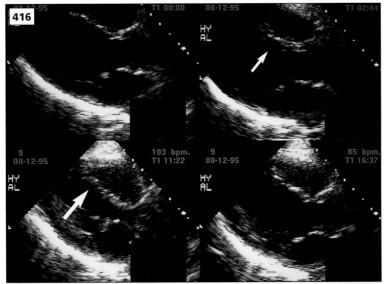

416, 417. In this quad-screen format the top left-hand image is at rest, the top right at low-dose dobutamine, the bottom left at peak stress, and the bottom right is taken during recovery. In this patient the posterior wall is clearly normal, thickening and becoming hypercontractile at peak stress. The anterior-septum increases in contractility at low-dose dobutamine (arrow) but with increasing cardiac workload becomes akinetic (large arrow). This is evidence of inducible ischemia in the left anterior descending coronary artery territory. The color-enhanced image confirms the anteroseptal akinesis (**417**, arrows). Color enhancement is probably of greater value in cases where changes in wall motion are more subtle.

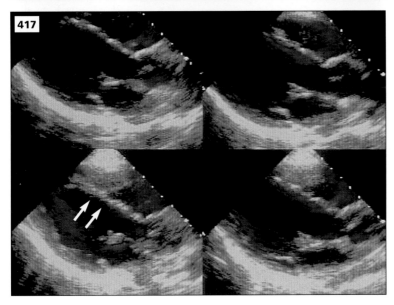

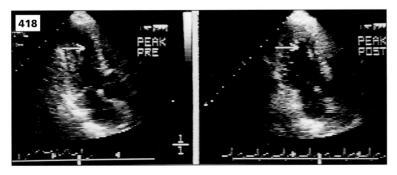

418. This patient had a left anterior descending coronary artery stenosis but very atypical chest pain and a non-diagnostic exercise stress test. Stress echocardiography reproduced his symptoms and he developed marked hypokinesis of the mid-anteroseptum at peak stress (left-hand image, arrow). Stress echocardiography was repeated post-angioplasty of a stenosis in the left anterior descending coronary artery and this time there is a normal response with endocardial movement and myocardial thickening evident at peak stress (right-hand image, arrow).

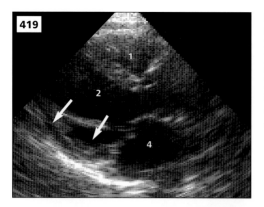

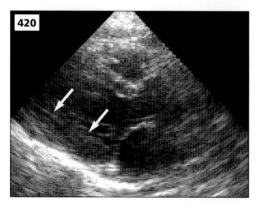

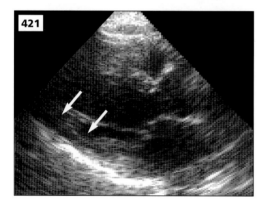

419–421. Improvement in myocardial function with low-dose dobutamine, indicative of viability of hibernating myocardium, may be subtle. In this sequence of images, the posterior wall is markedly hypokinetic at rest (arrows) (**419**). With low-dose dobutamine there is an increase in myocardial thickening (**420**), but the function of the posterior wall deteriorates with increases cardiac workload (**421**). This pattern indicates myocardial viability of this segment with underlying significant coronary obstructive disease. 1, RV; 2, LV; 4, LA.

Direct imaging of coronary arteries

In adults, it is possible occasionally to obtain echo-cardiographic images of the origins of the right and left coronary arteries.

In children, the coronary arteries can be imaged through much of their length; this is particularly important in those with anomalous coronary arteries and Kawasaki syndrome.

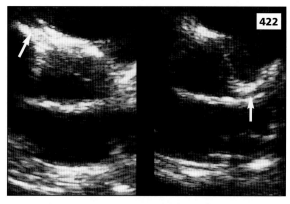

422. In this example, the right and left coronary arteries (arrows) are seen in short-axis views, just above the aortic valve.

- *Intravascular ultrasound has the major advantage over angiography as it details the anatomy not only of the arterial lumen, but also of the wall, which is the site of the atheromatous disease under examination.*

- *It is of particular use in:*
  - *(i) the apparently 'normal' vessel on angiography;*
  - *(ii) ensuring that there is adequate stent deployment; and*
  - *(iii) determining the nature of a plaque.*

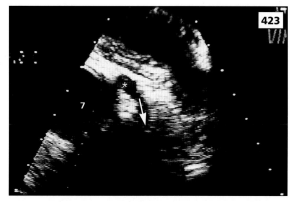

423. By transesophageal echocardiography, due to the closer proximity of the transducer with the great arteries, more detail can be seen but clinically important information is very infrequently obtained. In this case, both the origin of the left coronary artery (*) and left anterior descending (arrow) can be seen clearly. 7, AO.

The delivery of an ultrasound transducer into the lumen of an artery allows detailed examination of the nature of an arterial plaque. Intravascular ultrasound (IVUS) is particularly useful to ensure adequate deployment of intracoronary stents (**424–428**).

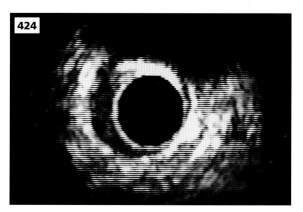

424. In this case, a calcified plaque is seen between 10 and 3 o'clock. The defect within the middle of the trace represents the shadow created by the catheter itself.

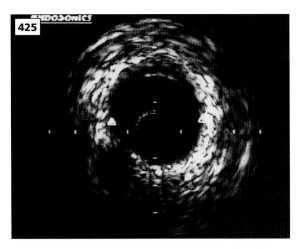

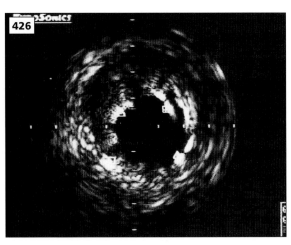

425. A left anterior descending artery proximal to the stenosis, the vessel diameter is 3.5 mm. There is soft plaque from 11 to 1 o'clock.

426. Partially deployed Palma–Schatz stent. The struts of the stent are not embedded into the arterial walls and are seen within the lumen. The measured transverse diameter is 2.7 mm.

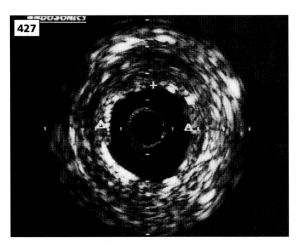

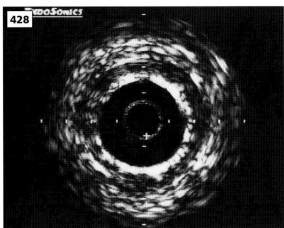

427. Proximal portion of stent almost completely deployed. The intimal surface is a little irregular and the cross-sectional shape is not circular.

428. Fully deployed Palma–Schatz stent. The cross-sectional shape is circular after high-pressure balloon dilatation and the diameter is 3.5 mm – the same as the reference vessel.

15 CARDIOMYOPATHIES

While the classification of cardiomyopathy into hypertrophic, dilated and restrictive was first introduced in the 1970s, it was not until the advances in echocardiography that such a differentiation could be clinically appreciated. The general classification is shown in *Table 15*. The diagnosis of dilated and hypertrophic cardiomyopathies is a simple one made on left ventricular cavity size and function and degree of left ventricular hypertrophy. The diagnosis of restrictive cardiomyopathy, either of idiopathic or a secondary form such as amyloidosis, is often much more difficult to confirm. Restrictive cardiomyopathies are often associated with small left ventricular cavities which are hypertrophied and associated with large atria. In such cases, the presence or absence of pericardial thickening to exclude constriction and an assessment of the degree of left ventricular hypertrophy is necessary for an etiologic diagnosis.

Hypertrophic Cardiomyopathy

In the diagnosis of hypertrophic cardiomyopathy it is probably best to divide these features into three separate groups: (i) those in whom there is a certain diagnosis; (ii) those in whom the diagnosis is relatively certain; and (iii) those in whom the diagnosis is uncertain. For a certain diagnosis, the presence of severe left ventricular hypertrophy, particularly affecting the ventricular septum or apex with evidence of left ventricular outflow tract obstruction, in the absence of a secondary cause, leads to a certain diagnosis. When there is moderate left ventricular hypertrophy or symmetric hypertrophy without a secondary cause or outflow tract obstruction, the diagnosis is fairly certain. In the presence of mild hypertrophy, which is symmetric and without outflow tract obstruction, the diagnosis is uncertain.

Table 15. Cardiomyopathies	
Hypertrophic	Idiopathic Hypertrophic cardiomyopathy Friedrich's ataxia
Dilated	Idiopathic End-stage ischemia/valvular/hypertension Chronic valve disease (mitral and aortic regurgitation) Post-viral Alcohol Post-partum Familial Adriamycin (dose related) Muscular dystrophies Thiamine deficiency Hemachromatosis
Restrictive and infiltrative	Idiopathic restrictive Infiltrations, e.g. amyloid Sarcoid Endomyocardial fibrosis Loefflers endocarditis Inherited infiltrations • glycogen storage disease • mucopolysaccharide storage diseases • Fabry's

It must be remembered that in the elderly it is not abnormal to have a subaortic septal bulge (sigmoid septum) and that this does not represent hypertrophic cardiomyopathy.

- *Careful examination of all the regions of the myocardium is necessary to diagnose the presence and distribution of abnormal muscle in hypertrophic cardiomyopathy.*
- *While the severity of left ventricular hypertrophy is a weak prognostic indicator, the echocardiogram predominantly yields diagnostic information.*

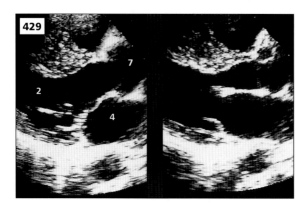

429. Parasternal long-axis view in systole and diastole showing a typical case of hypertrophic cardiomyopathy without left ventricular outflow tract obstruction. In this case there is considerable thickening of the ventricular septum (more than 2 cm) with a normal thickness posterior wall. This leads to asymmetric septal hypertrophy. The left ventricular outflow tract is widely patent with no muscle encroachment or anterior motion of the mitral valve in systole. In this case, the left atrium is of normal size. 2, LV; 4, LA; 7, AO.

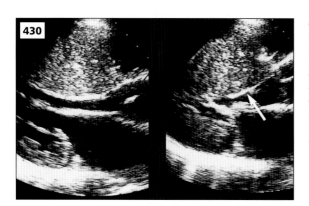

430. Parasternal long-axis view in severe hypertrophic cardiomyopathy. There is gross ventricular hypertrophy involving the septum and, to a much lesser extent, the posterior wall. In diastole, the left ventricular outflow tract is considerably narrowed due to encroachment of the septum. In systole, there is obstruction to the outflow tract by the anterior leaflet of the mitral valve (arrow) and by apposition of the papillary muscles to the septum. In such cases there may be outflow and mid-cavity left ventricular obstruction.

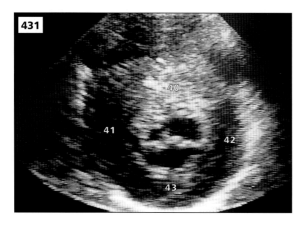

431. It is best to define the distribution of left ventricular hypertrophy on parasternal short-axis views. In this example at the level of the mitral valve, there is mild hypertrophy of the posterior and free walls of the left ventricle. However, there is considerable thickening of the anterior (40) and posterior (41) ventricular septum. This is the most common distribution of left ventricular hypertrophy found in hypertrophic cardiomyopathy. The distribution may be localized at the anterior septum (40) alone, posterior septum (41), free wall (42), and, less commonly, the apex of the ventricle. 43, Posterior wall.

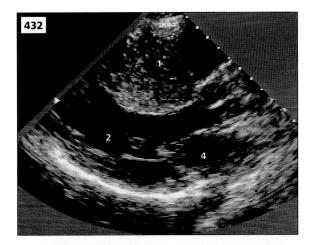

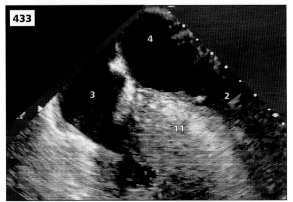

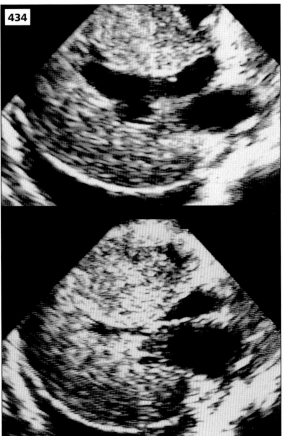

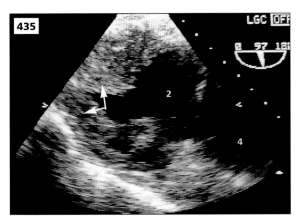

432, 433. To further define the nature and distribution of left ventricular hypertrophy, transesophageal echocardiography may be useful. In this parasternal transthoracic long-axis view, gross hypertrophy of the ventricular septum is seen with a relatively normal-thickness posterior wall (**432**). By transesophageal echocardiography, the hypertrophy of the septum (11) is seen to extend from below the mitral ring to the apex (**433**). 1, RV; 2, LV; 3, RA; 4, LA; 11, IVS.

434. The other forms of hypertrophic cardiomyopathy with symmetric and apical involvement predominantly, are less commonly found. Symmetric distribution of left ventricular hypertrophy is more common in young patients. In this case, the myocardium is hypertrophied to an equal degree in the ventricular septum, posterior wall, and free wall. The left ventricular cavity is tiny and, in systole, almost completely disappears. Such patients have very considerable outflow tract and intracavity gradients. 2, LV; 4, LA; 7, AO.

435. Apical left ventricular hypertrophy in hypertrophic cardiomyopathy is difficult to image by transthoracic echocardiography. In this case transesophageal echocardiography (transgastric longitudinal view) readily shows the extent of apical left ventricular hypertrophy (arrows) and relative sparing of the base. 2, LV; 4, LA.

Assessment of left ventricular outflow tract obstruction

There are various proposed mechanisms of intracavity and left ventricular outflow tract obstruction in hypertrophic cardiomyopathy. They include systolic anterior motion of the mitral valve, apposition of the papillary muscles (and their abnormal insertion) to the ventricular septum, and obliteration of the cavity.

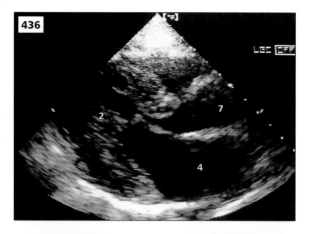

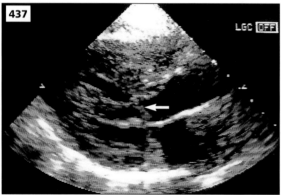

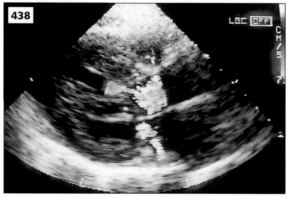

436–438. There is little thickening of the anterior leaflet of the mitral valve in diastole (**436**), but in systole it can be seen to move anteriorly towards the thickened ventricular septum (**437**) (arrow). There is almost complete apposition of the anterior leaflet of the mitral valve and septum, so the degree of obstruction may be considerable. Color flow localizes the obstruction to this site (**438**). 2, LV; 4, LA; 7, AO.

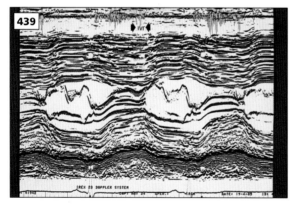

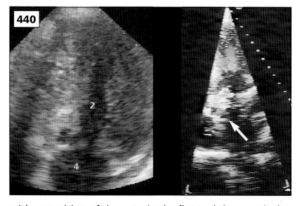

439, 440. Because of the speed of movement of the anterior leaflet of the mitral valve when it is drawn forward by the Venturi effect of the rapid initial ejection of blood, it may well not be seen while at the slow scanning speed of two-dimensional echocardiography. It is often better seen by M-mode echocardiography, with its higher frame rate. In this example (**439**), there is definite evidence of anterior motion of the mitral valve with apposition of the anterior leaflet and the ventricular septum. The left ventricular outflow tract obstruction may be due to encroachment by the ventricular septum. The obstruction may, however, be mid-cavity (**440**). There is severe symmetric left ventricular hypertrophy and in systole, the color flow abnormalities are seen within the ventricular cavity (arrow), and with continuous-wave Doppler the velocity exceeds 5 m/s (arrow). 2, LV; 4, LA.

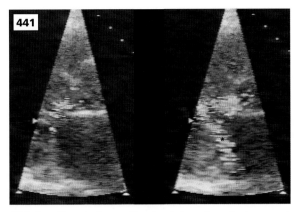

441. Systolic anterior motion leads to valvar displacement and occasionally mitral regurgitation. In this example, in early systole, a turbulent jet is seen in the outflow tract due to the development of obstruction (arrow). As systole progresses the gradient rises and there is a jet of mitral regurgitation (*). 4, LA.

In a patient with left ventricular hypertrophy, dehydration or inotropic support may lead to a dynamic intracavitary gradient.

- *Left ventricular outflow tract obstruction may be very ephemeral and only observed under particular loading conditions and imaging in one plane.*
- *It is imperative to search for causes of fixed or membranous subaortic obstruction in patients with left ventricular outflow tract obstruction.*
- *Patients suitable for myectomy need significant left ventricular outflow tract obstruction and hypertrophy preferably localized to the upper septum.*

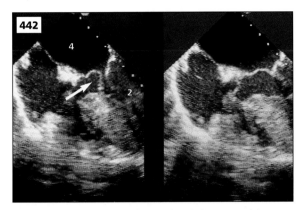

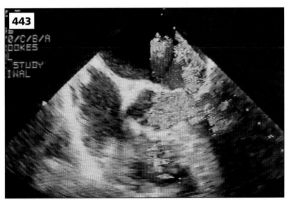

442, 443. Outflow tract obstruction in hypertrophic cardiomyopathy may be examined using transesophageal echocardiography if the transthoracic images are suboptimal. In this example, there is ventricular septal hypertrophy with a narrowed ventricular outflow tract. In systole left, there is anterior motion of the anterior

leaflet of the mitral valve coming into apposition with the ventricular septum (arrow). In systole, there is both turbulent forward blood flow from this area due to left ventricular outflow tract obstruction and mitral regurgitation. 2, LV; 4, LA.

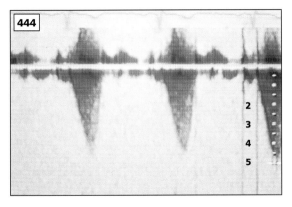

444. Continuous-wave recording of left ventricular outflow tract obstruction is best carried out from the apex. In this example, there is a large gradient across the left ventricular outflow tract. The typical shape of these traces is due to an initial flow – suggesting mitral regurgitation – and then a slowly rising 'scimitar-shape' gradient of dynamic left ventricular outflow tract obstruction.

Left Ventricular Hypertrophy

While the diagnosis of hypertrophic cardio-myopathy rests on the demonstration of left ventricular hypertrophy (LVH) in the absence of a cause, most patients with myocardial thickening and increased mass will have clinical evidence for its origin.

The most common cause for LVH is hypertension. The demonstration of increased myocardial mass in such patients carries an independent risk for the development of all forms of cardiovascular disease. The degree of hypertrophy is only poorly related to isolated measurements of blood pressure – especially when treated – but correlates better with long-term estimates of hypertension. Tight control of hypertension will lead to regression of myocardial hypertrophy. There is a large number of causes of primary and secondary left ventricular hypertrophy which are dealt with under the specific sections.

Hypertension is the most common cause of hypertrophy and is only poorly related to isolated measurements of resting blood pressure.

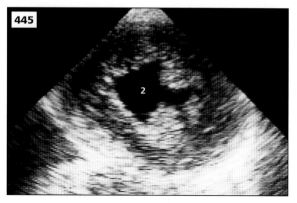

445. Parasternal short-axis of severe symmetric left ventricular hypertrophy in a patient with long-standing, poorly controlled hypertension. There are no specific features to distinguish this form of hypertrophy from any other, and knowledge of the clinical status of the patient is essential. 2, LV.

Dilated Cardiomyopathy

The demonstration of a dilated and poorly contracting left ventricle does not lead to an etiologic diagnosis. Dilated cardiomyopathy may be the end-stage of a number of disease processes. If there are no obvious primary or secondary causes, the usual diagnosis is one of idiopathic dilated cardiomyopathy. Except in unusual circumstances, one cannot differentiate this from end-stage ischemic heart disease, hypertensive heart disease, and specific heart muscle disorders.

The finding of a dilated and poorly contracting left ventricle gives no information concerning its etiology.

446–453 *opposite.* Sequence of echocardiograms in a patient with dilated cardiomyopathy of relatively recent onset. There is a dilated and poorly contracting left ventricle. The myocardium appears thin without compensatory hypertrophy which is thought to be a prognostic factor for impaired survival. The pericardium is thin and there is no fluid seen. Color flow imaging shows there to be a broad jet of central mitral regurgitation due to dilatation of the annulus and failure of valvar coaptation. The left atrium is moderately enlarged, as is the right ventricle. The left ventricle in this example remains relatively ellipsoid and has not, as yet, become spherical in shape. Apical color-flow imaging shows there to be a jet of mitral regurgitation arising centrally because of the dilated mitral annulus, as well as a shorter jet of tricuspid regurgitation. Doppler interrogation of the tricuspid jet shows there to be a ventricular–atrial gradient of 2–3 m/s, suggesting that pulmonary artery pressure is normal. In this example there is rapid atrial fibrillation and the variation in pressure gradient is readily seen (**453**). It is best to assess left ventricular size and function by M-mode echocardiographic measurements. 1, RV; 2, LV; 3, RA; 4, LA; 7, AO.

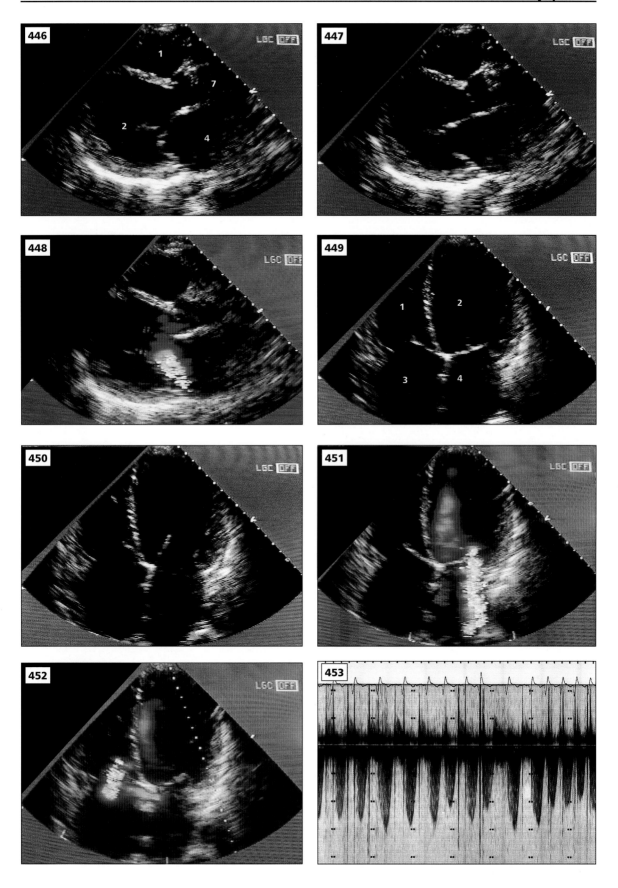

> *The right ventricle is considered to be dilated if it is the same size or bigger than the left ventricle. Right ventricular dilatation may be due to:*
> - *Dilated cardiomyopathy.*
> - *Left-to-right shunt.*
> - *Pulmonary hypertension:*
>   - *mitral stenosis*
>   - *pulmonary embolic disease*
>   - *primary*
> - *Tricuspid regurgitation/pulmonary regurgitation.*
> - *Right ventricular infarction.*

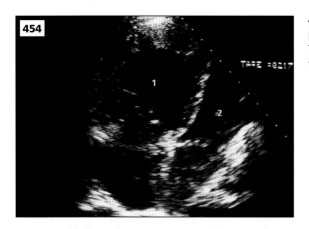

454. Much less commonly, dilated cardiomyopathy may predominantly involve the right ventricle. In this example, the right ventricle is much more enlarged than the left and there is laminated apical thrombus. 1, RV; 2, LV.

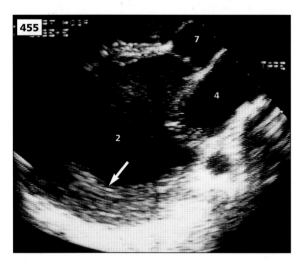

455. While it is generally supposed that viral myocarditis is the predetermined factor in idiopathic dilated cardiomyopathy, there is currently little evidence to support this for the majority of cases. However, occasionally viral infection is confirmed, and in this example there was rapid onset of ventricular dilatation with a thickened and edematous appearance to the posterior ventricular wall (arrows). The pericardium is also involved, in this case of myopericarditis. 2, LV; 4, LA; 7, AO.

Idiopathic Restrictive Cardiomyopathy

In a patient with heart failure and normal left ventricular contraction, the diagnosis of restrictive cardiomyopathy or constrictive pericarditis should be considered. These may be differentiated by the Doppler inflow patterns (rapid initial filling) and the absence of pericardial thickening on echocardiography, CT-, or MRI-scanning. The echocardiographic features of restrictive cardiomyopathy are of small – often hypertrophied – left and right ventricles, with gross dilatation of the atria. The atria often take on a rather spherical appearance and may have thrombus sited within them. Left ventricular motion has a jerky appearance.

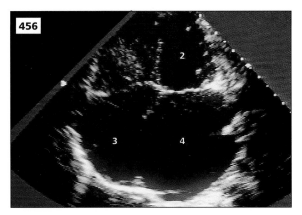

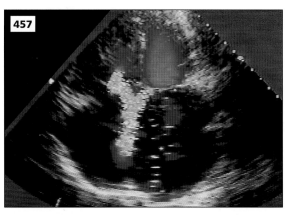

456, 457. Mild restrictive cardiomyopathy showing an elongated and non-hypertrophied left ventricle. The atria are considerably enlarged. The right ventricle is small and there is no conspicuous hypertrophy. Mitral and tricuspid regurgitation are common in these conditions. The jets of regurgitant flow can clearly be seen by color flow and, because of their angulation, by mid-systole tend to run down each side of the intra-atrial septum (**457**). 2, LV; 3, RA; 4, LA.

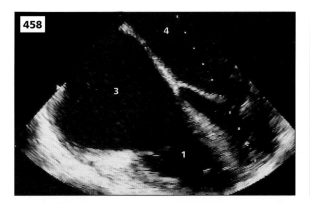

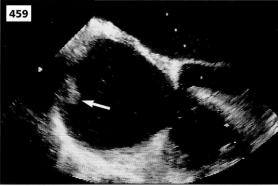

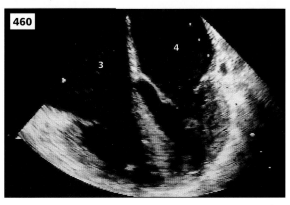

458–460. Transesophageal echocardiography may be particularly useful in determining the presence of right atrial thrombus. In this young woman, who presented with pulmonary emboli and atrial fibrillation, there is gross atrial enlargement (particularly the right) which is seen by superior angulation of the transducer. There is thrombus on the posterior wall of the right atrium (arrow). There is, in addition, in this example, moderate left ventricular hypertrophy. 1, RV; 3, RA; 4, LA.

Amyloid heart disease

In the West, with its aging population, amyloid heart disease is a not uncommon form of heart failure. This may be recognized by a non-dilated, markedly hypertrophied and poorly contracting left ventricle. While some suggest that the echocardiographic texture of the myocardium is abnormal, this is often an unhelpful sign in the elderly. Left ventricular inflow is abnormal, the E-wave becomes reduced, and the A-wave becomes dominant. This is a reflection of abnormal left ventricular properties in diastole.

The progression of cardiac amyloid can be very rapid and an initially normal echo can show typical features within a few months.

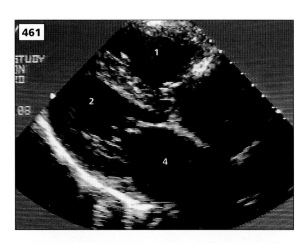

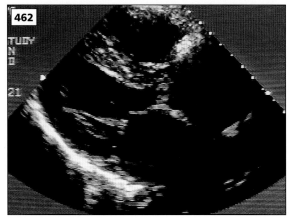

461, 462. Systolic and diastolic frames of a patient with cardiac amyloidosis. There is moderate left ventricular hypertrophy with poor contraction. Atrial enlargement is often considerable and there may often be a pericardial effusion. The aortic valve may become thickened and occasionally significantly stenosed. The appearance of the thickened myocardium in amyloid may be abnormal. 1, RV; 2, LV; 4, LA.

Echocardiographic features of amyloid include:

- *Symmetric left ventricular hypertrophy.*
- *Poor left ventricular contraction without dilatation.*
- *The myocardium may have a speckled appearance.*
- *Right ventricular hypertrophy.*
- *Valvular thickening.*
- *Biatrial enlargement.*

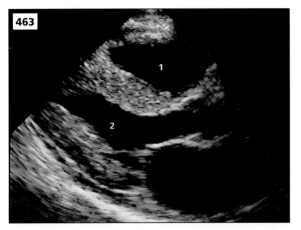

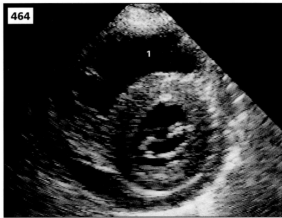

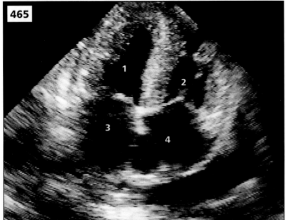

463–466. Parasternal long- and short-axis views in a patient with cardiac amyloidosis, demonstrating concentric left ventricular hypertrophy. The apical four-chamber view confirms biventricular involvement with relatively normal cavity size. The mitral and tricuspid valves are mildly thickened. This patient also had pericardial and pleural effusions. The left ventricular M-mode shows poor contraction of the left ventricle. 1, RV; 2, LV; 3, RA; 4, LA.

Differentiation of restrictive cardiomyopathy from constrictive pericarditis is shown in *Table 16*.

Table 16.
Differentiation of restrictive cardiomyopathy from constrictive pericarditis

	Restrictive	Constrictive
Pericardium	Normal	May be thickened
Atria	Large	Normal
LVH	Yes	No
Ejection fraction	⇓	Normal
LV filling velocities	No variation with respiration	⇓ with inspiration
SVC flow		
⇑ reversal	in inspiration	in expiration
forward flow	predominantly diastolic	variable pattern

Endomyocardial fibrosis

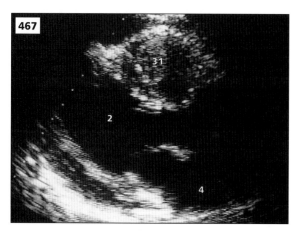

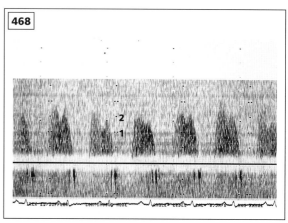

467, 468. Endomyocardial fibrosis is rare in the West, though a common condition in tropical climates when associated with eosinophilic diseases. Echocardiographically, the features may be of restrictive cardiomyopathy, though the involvement of the endocardium often leads to bright reflectance from this area. Its features otherwise resemble restrictive cardiomyopathy, though there is a high propensity to thrombus formation in ventricular cavities which may involve the atrioventricular valves. Contraction of the fibrous tissue is common and may lead to mitral and tricuspid regurgitation. Thrombus formation (31), as in this example in the right ventricle (**467**) may be associated with valvar involvement and lead to tricuspid stenosis (**468**). 2, LV; 4, LA.

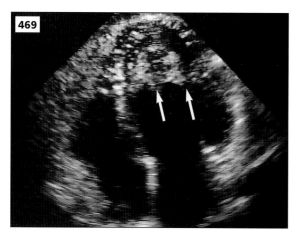

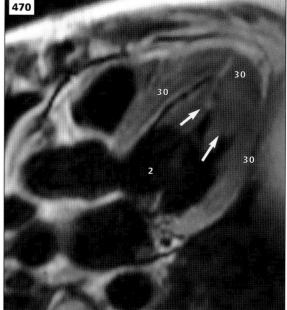

469, 470. An apical four-chamber view in a patient with endomyocardial fibrosis (**469**). There are echogenic deposits obliterating the left ventricular apex and extending to the base of the papillary muscles (arrows). Superimposed thrombus formation occurs frequently. Extension of the endocardial thickening can lead to involvement of the mitral valve with severe regurgitation. An MRI scan in this patient confirms that the apical deposits are due to marked endocardial thickening as shown by the lighter grey area (arrows) compared with the denser normal myocardium (30) (**470**). 2, LV.

16 SINUS OF VALSALVA ANEURYSM

A sinus of Valsalva aneurysm, particularly when it ruptures, is an important differential diagnostic feature of chest pain and aortic regurgitation and continuous murmurs. Prior to rupture, it may lead to obstruction of the tricuspid valve or the right ventricle. The aneurysm may arise anywhere within the circumference of the aorta.

The presence of turbulent blood flow, shown by color-flow Doppler, around the aortic root should raise the suspicion of either a sinus of Valsalva fistula or a subaortic ventricular septal defect. Careful scanning to identify the site of shunt as being above or below the aortic valve is required.

471, 472. Short-axis view in systole and diastole in a patient with a bicuspid aortic valve, dilatation of the aortic root due to Marfan's syndrome, and an unruptured sinus of Valsalva aneurysm (arrow). This is arising near the origin of the left coronary artery and moves with the cardiac cycle. 7, AO.

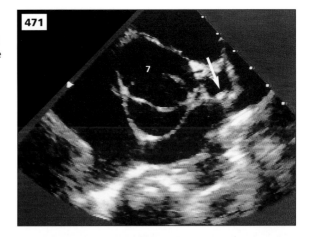

- *Sinus of Valsalva aneurysms involve the right coronary sinus in approximately 70% of cases, the non-coronary sinuses in about 25%, and the left coronary sinus in only 5%.*

- *When a sinus ruptures, the resultant echo findings are determined by the size of the shunt, by the speed at which the shunt develops, and by the chamber which receives the shunt flow.*

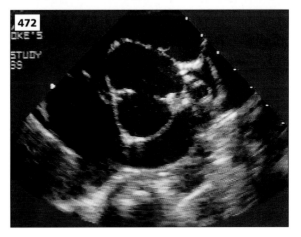

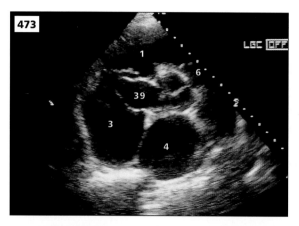

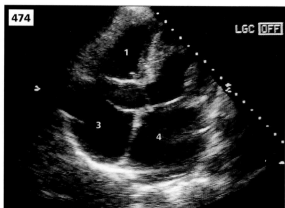

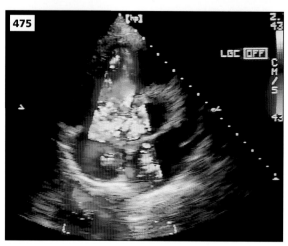

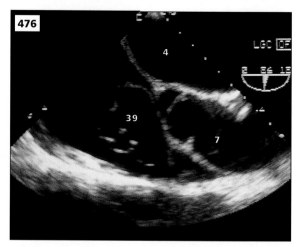

473–477. This shows a well-defined aneurysm (39, seen by short- and long-axis views) arising near the origin of the right coronary artery. The aneurysm extends beneath the tricuspid annulus and has ruptured into the right atrium. The rupture of these aneurysms – to become a fistula – is usually a catastrophic event and leads to flow between the aorta and any other intracardiac structure, but most commonly the right ventricle or right atrium. The fistulous communication is shown by color flow (**475**). Transesophageal echo in the same patient shows the extensive nature of the aneurysm (**476**) with flow (**477**) into the right atrium. 1, RV; 3, RA; 4, LA; 6, PA; 7, AO.

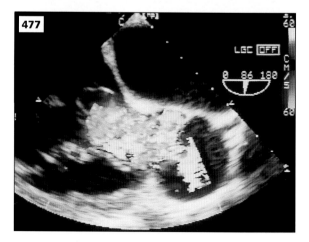

17 CONGENITAL HEART DISEASE

The introduction of echocardiography has allowed the bedside diagnosis of many forms of congenital heart disease. The range of possible congenital heart disease is very wide and we intend to demonstrate only those forms seen commonly in adults.

Ventricular Septal Defect

Ventricular septal defects are common congenital abnormalities and may occur in isolation or as part of a more complex anomaly. Anatomically, ventricular septal defects are divided at the level of the crista supraventricularis into supracrystal and infracrystal defects. Supracrystal defects are also termed infundibular and occur just below the pulmonary valve. Infracrystal defects are divided into membranous (subaortic), muscular, and inlet septal defects.

The most common finding in the examination of patients with small ventricular septal defects is an abnormal jet of color flow, even if the defect is not imaged directly. Some apical defects may only been seen by unusual angulation of the transducer.

The peak jet velocity in ventricular septal defect measured by continuous-wave Doppler will allow measurement of the pressure difference between the left and right ventricles. Subtraction of the pressure difference from the cuff systolic pressure will give right ventricular pressure, and pulmonary arterial systolic pressure may be calculated in the absence of right ventricular outflow obstruction.

Care must be taken to record the peak jet velocity. A low jet velocity would suggest pulmonary hypertension, but may be due to poor scanning technique missing the true peak velocity; a high jet velocity must mean a large pressure differential between the ventricles, and so excludes pulmonary hypertension.

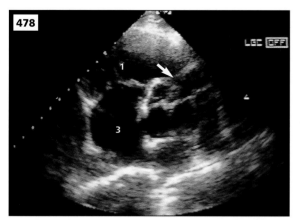

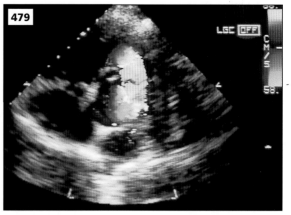

478, 479. A supracrystal (infundibular) ventricular septal defect is imaged is shown on this parasternal short-axis view at the level of the aortic valve (arrows). The pulmonary valve is also thickened. 1, RV; 3, RA.

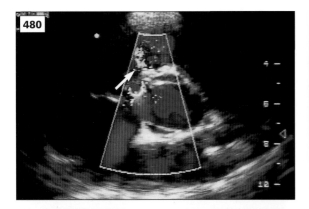

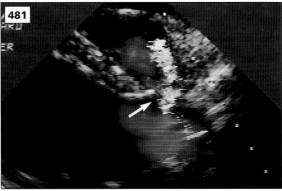

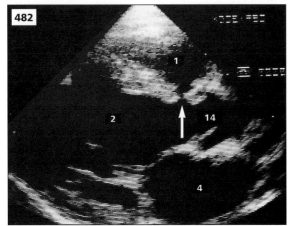

480–482. The parasternal short-axis view at the aortic valve level demonstrates color flow from left-to-right through a membranous ventricular septal defect (arrow) (**480**). In this example of a parasternal long-axis view, an abnormal color-flow jet is shown in the membranous ventricular outflow tract (arrow) (**481**). There is an abnormal turbulent area on the left ventricular side of the defect due to flow convergence. As the defects become larger, they are often visualized directly (arrow) (**482**). All available windows need to be imaged before excluding the diagnosis of a ventricular septal defect. Ventricular septal defects can occur in any part of the ventricular septum from subaortic, subtricuspid, inflow, and muscular. 1, RV; 2, LV; 4, LA; 14, AoV.

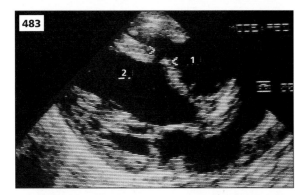

483. This example is a mid-septal muscular defect of moderate size; such defects are often difficult to image because they are sited towards the apex. 1, RV; 2, LV.

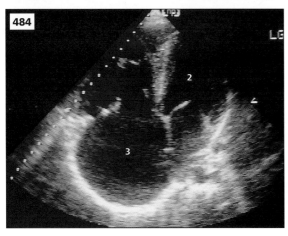

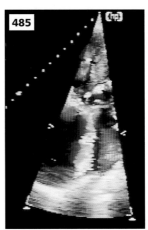

484, 485. As the defect enlarges there will be dilatation of the right ventricle and right atrium, often associated with a rising pulmonary artery pressure and tricuspid regurgitation. 2, LV; 3, RA.

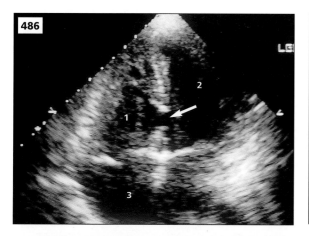

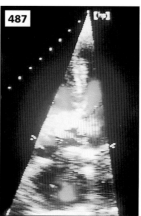

486, 487. The apical four-chamber demonstrates a mid-septal muscular defect (**486**) (arrow) with left-to-right shunting on color flow (**487**). 1, RV; 2, LV; 3, RA.

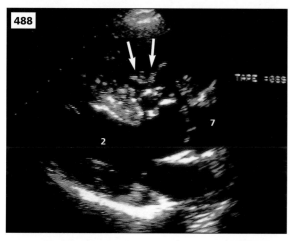

488. Ventricular septal defects in the membranous outflow tract tend to close spontaneously by the application of the septal leaflet of the tricuspid valve to the defect. This may produce a very curious pattern with reduplication of valve tissue, possibly with aneurysmal dilatation and flow patterns around it (arrows). 2, LV; 7, AO.

If the right ventricle is dilated and right-sided flow velocities increased, a shunt is likely to be significant.

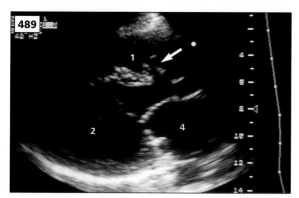

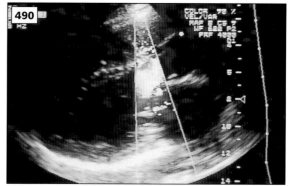

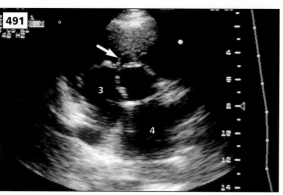

489–491. Membranous ventricular septal aneurysms develop as part of the natural process of closure of ventricular septal defects. The initial formation of a ventricular septal aneurysm is frequently associated with partial closure of the defect with a decrease in left-to-right shunt. A membranous ventricular septal aneurysm is illustrated in this parasternal long-axis view (arrow) (**489**). The color-flow image shows there is still some left-to-right shunting through the defect (**490**). The thin-walled aneurysm is seen protruding into the right ventricular cavity on the parasternal short-axis view (arrow) (**491**). 1, RV; 2, LV; 3, RA; 4, LA.

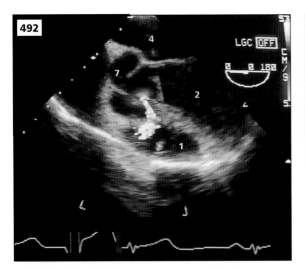

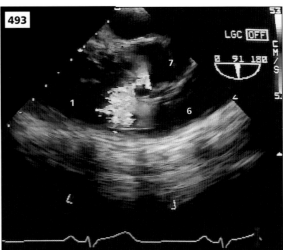

492, 493. Transesophageal echocardiography may demonstrate the defect when inadequately imaged by transthoracic echocardiography. In this case, transverse and longitudinal views show a subaortic membranous ventricular septal defect without evidence of right ventricular dilatation. Determining the magnitude of shunting can be inferred by the size of the right ventricle. Small defects tend to have a normal right ventricle and, as the magnitude of the shunt increases, so does the ventricular size. The color-flow maps have flow convergence and a high velocity. 1, RV; 2, LV; 4, LA; 6, PA; 7, AO.

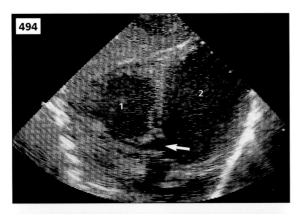

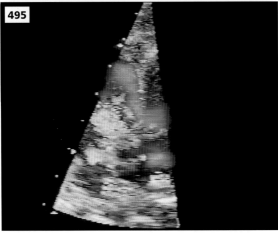

494, 495. Ventricular septal defects do not necessarily communicate between left and right ventricles: although uncommon, in the Gerbode type, the defect may be between the left ventricle and the right atrium. This may be clearly demonstrated by ultrasound, though occasionally the flow may be on both sides of the tricuspid valve. In this subcostal view in a child the defect is seen to open into the right atrium and that is the exit of the color flow turbulence. 1, RV; 2, LV.

The degree of shunting may be determined from the ratio of pulmonary to aortic stroke volume.

Pulmonary stroke volume (PSV) is derived from:
PSV = Area × Velocity Time Integral
Pulmonary diameter is measured at the annulus and area calculated from the formula Area = (πr^2)
Velocity time integral is measured by placing a pulsed Doppler sample volume at the same level and averaging the area under the curve for 5 cycles

Aortic stroke volume (ASV) is derived from:
ASV = Area × Velocity Time Integral
The left ventricular outflow tract diameter is measured on a parasternal long axis view and area calculated from the formula Area = (πr^2)

A pulsed Doppler sample volume is placed at the same level to measure the velocity time integral

The ratio of aortic to pulmonary flow is valid for shunt estimation in atrial septal defects and ventricular septal defects, providing that there is no turbulent flow in the pulmonary valve orifice. The assessment of shunting in patent ductus arteriosus is more complicated, as more than systemic flow passes through the aortic valve and less then pulmonary flow passes through the pulmonary valve. In these circumstances systemic and pulmonary flow should be measured at the mitral and tricuspid valves.

496. Long-standing large ventricular septal defects may develop the Eisenmenger reaction. In this example, there is gross hypertrophy of the right ventricle and of the right side of the ventricular septum. This may give the erroneous diagnosis of asymmetric septal hypertrophy as the posterior left ventricular wall is of normal thickness. 1, RV; 2, LV.

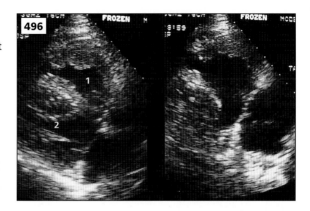

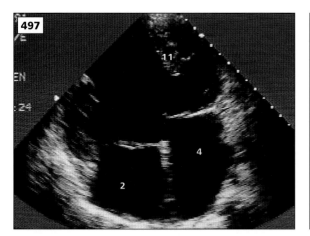

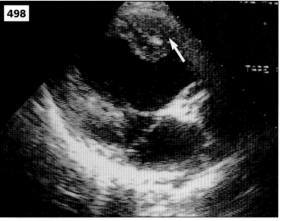

497, 498. Univentricular heart is the demonstration of a relative or complete absence of the ventricular septum. These patients always have systemic right ventricular pressures and the pulmonary artery pressure depends on the presence of pulmonary stenosis. It may be associated with other abnormalities, including transposition of the great arteries. In this example there is a vestigial ventricular septum. More commonly, there is an outflow rudimentary chamber, in this case lying anteriorly (arrow) (**498**). 2, LV; 4, LA; 11, IVS.

Atrial Septal Defect

Atrial septal defects are classified on the basis of their position in the septum and their embryologic origin. There are four types – ostium primum, ostium secundum, sinus venosus, and coronary sinus. Atrial septal defects are most commonly of the secundum type (70%) and are located in the region of the fossa ovalis. These defects occur as a result of the incomplete development of the septum secundum.

If a patient has paradoxical septal motion with right ventricular and right atrial volume overload, atrial septal defect must be actively excluded by all imaging modalities, particularly transesophageal echocardiography. It is important to examine the pulmonary venous drainage. Imaging and color flow may enable this directly. Transesophageal echocardiography is particularly useful for determining the sites of pulmonary venous drainage.

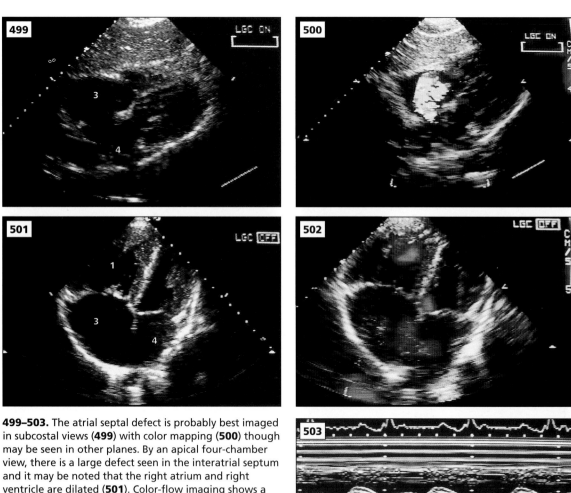

499–503. The atrial septal defect is probably best imaged in subcostal views (**499**) with color mapping (**500**) though may be seen in other planes. By an apical four-chamber view, there is a large defect seen in the interatrial septum and it may be noted that the right atrium and right ventricle are dilated (**501**). Color-flow imaging shows a broad, low velocity jet of laminar blood flow across the interatrial septum (**502**). This suggests that the defect is of hemodynamic importance. The classic M-mode feature of this condition is paradoxical septal motion (**503**). 1, RV; 3, RA; 4, LA.

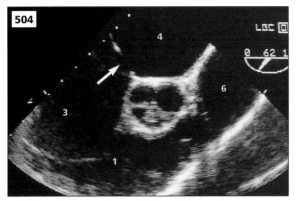

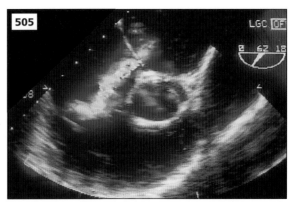

504, 505. Transesophageal echocardiography may demonstrate an atrial septal defect not visualized by other techniques. In this case, a small defect is seen without enlargement of the right atrium by a short-axis transesophageal echo (**504**). Color-flow Doppler demonstrates a narrow, non-laminar jet, suggesting a small defect (**505**). There is thickening of the aortic valve. 1, RV; 3, RA; 4, LA; 6, PA.

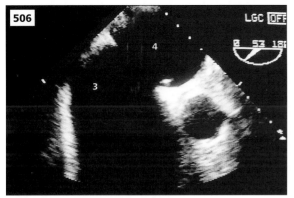

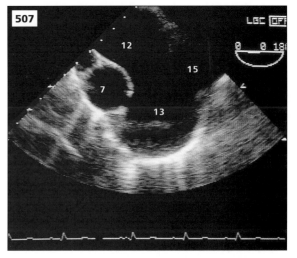

506, 507. If the defect is very large, even by transesophageal echo none of the secundum septum is seen (**506**). The main pulmonary artery (13) in this patient was considerably enlarged (**507**). 3, RA; 4, LA; 7, AO; 12, RPA; 13, MPA; 15, LPA.

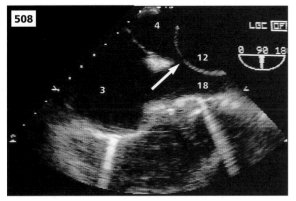

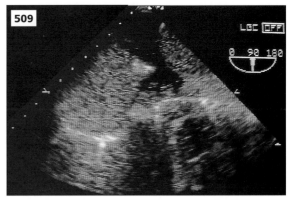

508, 509. Sinus venosus defects constitute 6–8% of atrial septal defects and the majority involve the superior vena cava. They are frequently associated with anomalous drainage of the right upper pulmonary vein. A sinus venosus defect is difficult to diagnose by transthoracic echo in adults, but by transesophageal echo is characteristically seen at the junction of the superior vena cava and right atrium (arrow) (note the enlarged right pulmonary artery). Color-flow mapping, or in this case right heart contrast injection, demonstrates contrast enhancement of the right atrium, superior vena cava, and pulmonary artery and a negative defect in the superior vena cava from the left-to-right shunt (**509**). 3, RA; 4, LA; 18, SVC; 12, RPA.

Primum atrial septal defect

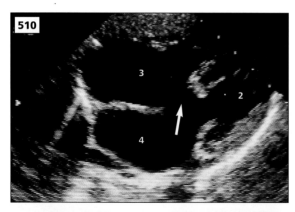

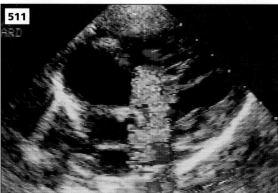

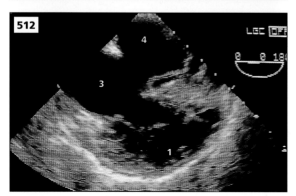

510–512. In contrast to the secundum defect, which is in the region of the foramen ovale, the primum defect lies lower in the atrial septum above the atrioventricular valves and comprises about 20% of atrial septal defects. Ostium primum defects result from incomplete fusion of the septum primum with the endocardial cushions and are considered a partial form of an atrioventricular canal. They are readily demonstrated by echocardiography. Subcostal imaging shows the defect (arrow) clearly with an intact secundum septum (**510**). In this example, the atrioventricular valves appear normal and there was no evidence of a ventricular septal defect. Color flow shows turbulent blood flow crossing from left to right atrium (**511**). Transesophageal echo in a transverse plane shows a large primum defect without a ventricular component; there is mild right ventricular enlargement and hypertrophy (**512**). 1, RV; 2, LV; 3, RA; 4, LA.

Atrioventricular Septal Defect

Primum atrial septal defect may coexist with a ventricular septal defect, which may be of variable size. The association of primum atrial and ventricular septal defects is often found in combination with bridging of the atrioventricular valve leaflets. There may be insertion of the papillary muscles and chordae into the crest of the ventricular septum.

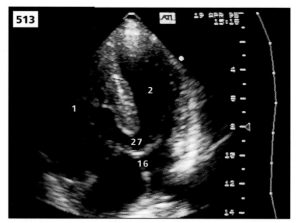

513. Apical four-chamber view: the primum atrial (16) and ventricular septal defects (27) can be seen with dilatation of the right atrium and right ventricle. The bridging nature of the anterior leaflet of the mitral valve is seen, but the insertion of chordae is not clear. 1, RV; 2, LV.

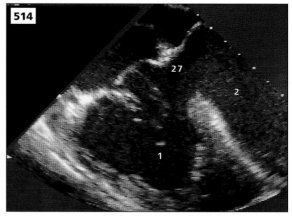

514. Transesophageal echocardiography may be useful for demonstrating the nature of the atrioventricular valves and their attachments. In this case, there is a large ventricular septal defect (27) with right ventricular enlargement and hypertrophy. There is a continuous atrioventricular valve with bridging of the anterior leaflet of the mitral valve. The tricuspid valve annulus is considerable dilated and this led to tricuspid regurgitation. Such information is particularly important before surgical repair. 1, RV; 2, LV.

Patent Ductus Arteriosus

In a child, the patent arterial duct may be readily seen by suprasternal imaging. In adults, this may be difficult but can often be picked up by the abnormal Doppler flow pattern in the left pulmonary artery. Shunt magnitude is probably best assessed semi-quantitatively by evidence of right ventricular and right atrial volume overload.

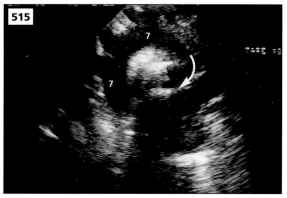

515. The arterial duct (arrow) can be seen in the suprasternal aortic arch view in a 4-year-old child. 7, AO.

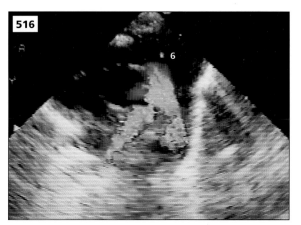

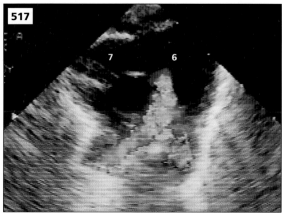

516, 517. The abnormal color-flow jet can be seen in the left pulmonary artery extending back into the main pulmonary artery. 6, PA; 7, AO.

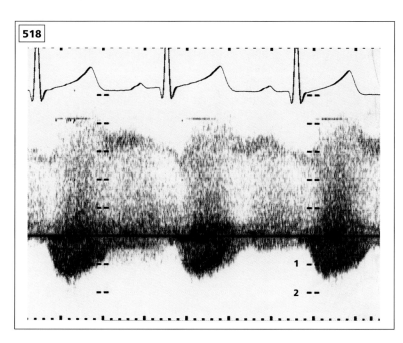

518. Continuous-wave Doppler across the patent ductus arteriosus gives a characteristic pattern with normal forward flow and continuous high-velocity flow in diastole.

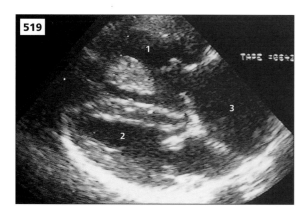

519. Although it is now unusual, the ductus arteriosus may be the cause of Eisenmenger syndrome. When this occurs there will be considerable right ventricular hypertrophy, though no abnormal flow may be seen across the duct because of balanced pressures. In this example, in the parasternal long-axis view, the tricuspid inflow is also seen; the right ventricle is grossly hypertrophied, and there is a huge muscle band within the hypertrophied papillary muscle. 1, RV; 2, LV; 3, RA.

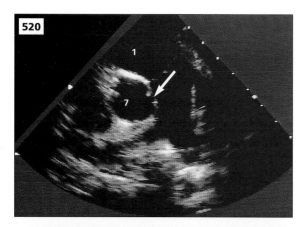

520–522. A patent ductus arteriosus needs to be differentiated from an aortic pulmonary window. This is a much less common diagnosis, but may have similar physical findings. The difference may be readily demonstrated by ultrasound. In this case, a defect is seen between the aorta and the main pulmonary artery (arrow). Abnormal color flow is shown in both short- (**521**) and long- (**522**) axis projections. 1, RV; 7, AO.

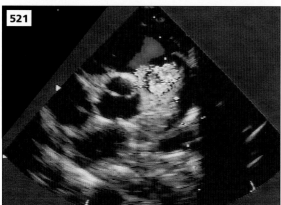

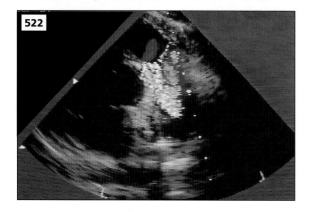

Pulmonary Stenosis

Cross-sectional imaging usually only gives long-axis views of the pulmonary valve and main pulmonary artery (usually this is all that is required). Multiplane transesophageal echocardiography allows more detailed examination of these structures.

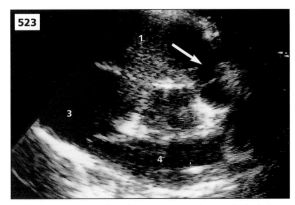

523. In patients with pulmonary stenosis, particularly in the young, there may be little to see other than doming and abnormal movement of a very slightly thickened valve (arrow). This is often best appreciated in parasternal short-axis views. 1, RV; 3, RA; 4, LA.

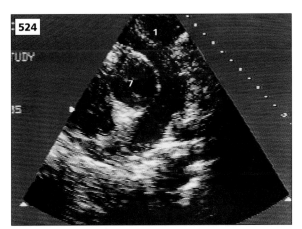

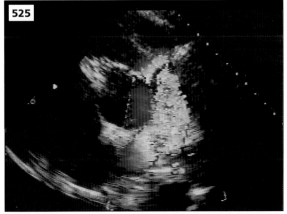

524, 525. The nature of the pulmonary stenosis may be apparent. In this example there is a dysplastic valve with a long-redundant leaflet with surplus tissue. Often, the valve appears to be inserted in a number of different sites. Although little may be seen of the valve itself, color-flow imaging shows very abnormal blood flow patterns within the pulmonary artery with flow convergence and an initial narrow jet (**525**). 1, RV; 7, AO.

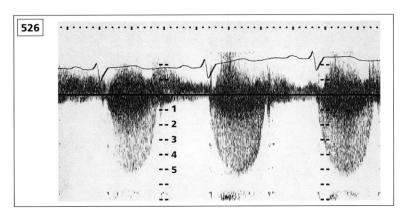

526. Continuous-wave Doppler will measure the degree of pulmonary valve obstruction; in this case over 5 m/s.

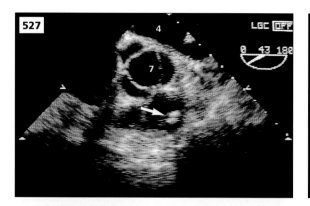

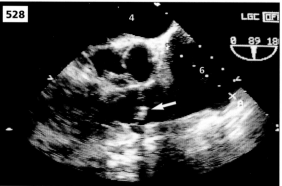

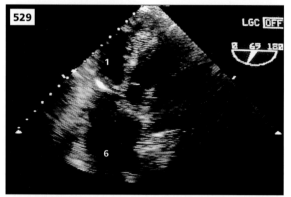

527–530. Despite the anterior position of the pulmonary valve it may be imaged well by transesophageal echocardiography. Short-axis (**527**) and longitudinal (**528**) views show a stenosed pulmonary valve (arrow) with post-stenotic aneurysmal dilatation evident on the longitudinal view (**528**). A low gastric view (**529**) allows correct alignment for Doppler interrogation, and in this example velocity across the pulmonary valve measured almost 4 m/s by continuous-wave Doppler (**530**). 1, RV; 4, LA; 6, PA; 7, AO.

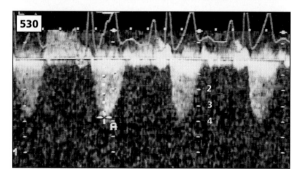

Tetralogy of Fallot

Tetralogy of Fallot is a combination of pulmonary stenosis and subaortic ventricular septal defect with overiding of the aorta. There is always associated right ventricular hypertrophy.

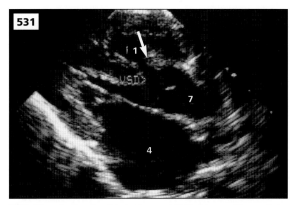

531. The diagnosis of tetralogy of Fallot is readily made by parasternal transthoracic echocardiography. The arrow shows the septal defect and aortic override. 1, RV; 4, LA; 7, AO.

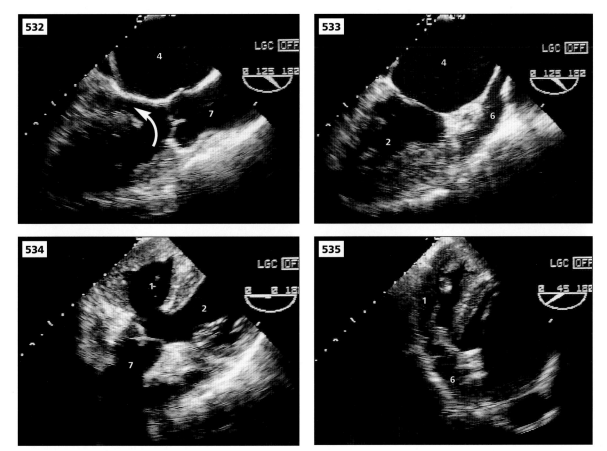

532–535. The features may be clarified by transesophageal echocardiography. A long-axis view demonstrates the overriding ascending aorta (**532**, arrow), and the subpulmonary obstruction and small pulmonary artery (**533**). A low gastric view allows assessment of the degree of septal override (**534**) and alignment for Doppler assessment of the pulmonary obstruction (**535**). 1, RV; 2, LV; 4, LA; 6, PA; 7, AO.

Truncus Arteriosus

The demonstration of a single trunk arising from the ventricles with the absence of a pulmonary artery leads to the diagnosis of truncus arteriosus. This needs to be differentiated from tetralogy of Fallot and is done so by determining the site of origin of the pulmonary arteries. These are often difficult to demonstrate by ultrasound, arising from the aorta in adult patients with truncus.

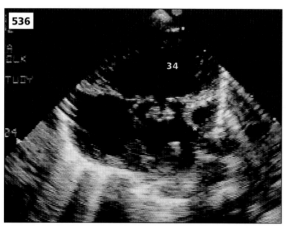

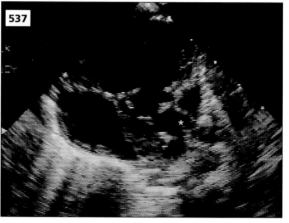

536, 537. Apical views showing a single trunk (*) arising from a combined ventricular cavity (34). The truncal valve is four-cuspid and often prolapses, which eventually leads to severe regurgitation. The pulmonary artery can be seen arising from the truncus.

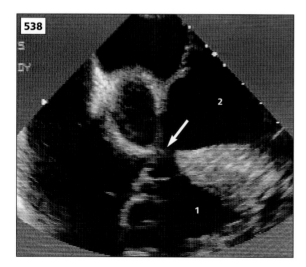

538. Transesophageal echocardiography may be useful for defining the nature of the truncus. In this case, the subaortic ventricular septal defect (arrow) is clearly seen with right ventricular hypertrophy. The trunk is considerably dilated and the pulmonary arteries arise anteriorly. 1, RV; 2, LV.

Miscellaneous

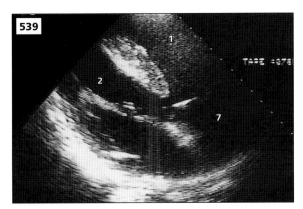

539. Truncus arteriosus needs to be differentiated from pulmonary atresia. This depends on demonstrating the pulmonary artery anatomy. In this example of pulmonary atresia with a ventricular septal defect, an overriding aorta is seen. In adults, the pulmonary arteries cannot usually be demonstrated by ultrasound. 1, RV; 2, LV; 7, AO.

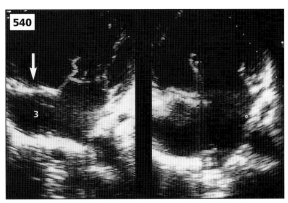

540. A tricuspid atresia is usually associated with a univentricular heart, transposition, or a large ventricular septal defect. It is readily demonstrated by cardiac ultrasound. The valve appears to be imperforate or occasionally hypoplastic (arrow). In this example, the mitral annulus is dilated and there is a common atrium. 3, RA.

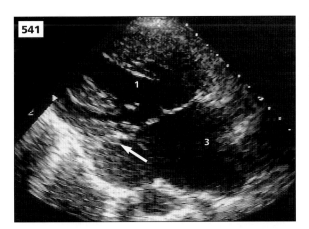

541. Mitral atresia is a less common defect but is again readily demonstrated. In this case, the area of the mitral valve is atretic (arrow) and the left ventricle is reduced to a 'slit-like' cavity seen posteriorly. The right ventricle is considerably hypertrophied. The atrial septum is present. 1, RV; 3, RA.

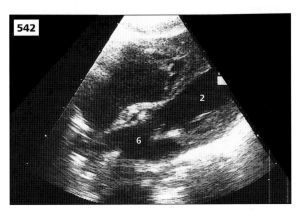

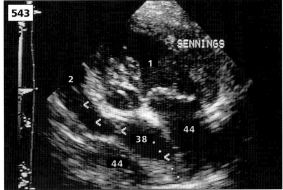

542, 543. Transposition of the great arteries may be seen by echocardiography, utilizing its ability to scan along the length of the great arteries, determining their nature and from which chamber they arise. The first illustration (**542**) shows the posterior cavity of the left ventricle giving rise to a branching vessel which is the pulmonary artery. Following an intra-atrial repair by a Senning procedure, the baffles can be clearly seen (**543**). 1, RV; 2, LV; 6, PA; 38, Systemic venous anastomosis; 44, Pulmonary venous anastomosis.

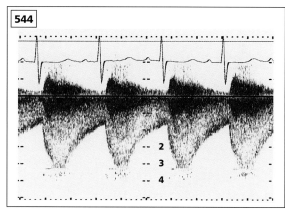

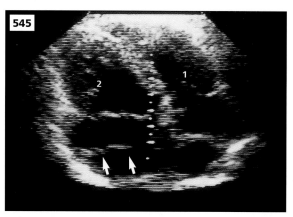

544. Coarctation of the aorta is difficult to image in adults but the continuous-wave Doppler pattern taken suprasternally is characteristic. There is continuous flow, maximum in systole, with a slow diastolic decline representing the collateral blood flow.

545. Cor triatriatum is a very rare form of mitral obstruction. It is occasionally seen as an isolated defect in adults. In this apical long-axis view a membrane is seen in the left atrium, separating the pulmonary venous origins from the mitral valve. The membrane in cor triatriatum (arrows) divides the atria above the atrial appendage and fossa ovalis. These features distinguish it from a supravalvular mitral ring. One or more openings permit the flow of blood from the pulmonary veins into the true left atrium. The size of the opening determines the degree of obstruction. 1, RV; 2, LV.

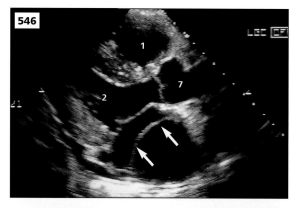

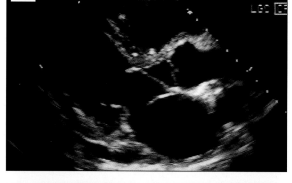

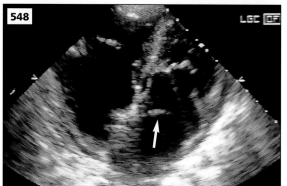

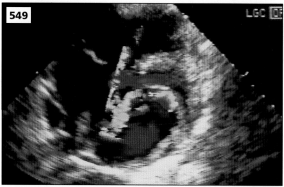

546–549. In this example, the membrane dividing the left atrium is apparent on the systolic and diastolic parasternal long-axis images (arrows) (**546, 547**). Assessment of obstruction, however, should be made on the apical four-chamber view (**548**) which allows measurement of the gradient across the membrane. The color-flow image (**549**) demonstrates an area of turbulence through the small, obstructive hole in the membrane. 1, RV; 2, LV; 7, AO.

Index

A bold number indicates an illustration of the item.